P9-CRF-102

quality and safety

Quality and Safety in Women's Health Care

Second Edition

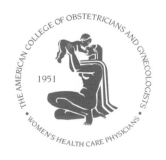

The American College of
Obstetricians and Gynecologists
Women's Health Care Physicians

Committee on Patient Safety and Quality Improvement (2008–2009)

John S. Wachtel, MD, *Chair*
Michele G. Curtis, MD, *Vice Chair*
Deborah A. Bartz, MD
Kenneth E. Brown, MD
Susan T. Haas, MD, MSc
Carol A. Keohane, RN
Larry Rand, MD
Larry L. Veltman, MD
Patrice M. Weiss, MD
Daniel J. Witkowski, MD
William H. Barth Jr, MD
Philip J. Diamond, MD

Phillip J. Goldstein, MD
John P. Keats, MD
Carol W. Saffold, MD
Paul A. Gluck, MD
R. Rima Jolivet, MSN, CNM, MPH
  (American College of Nurse–
  Midwives)
Paul J. Reiss, MD, FAAFP
  (American Academy of Family
  Physicians)
Stanley Zinberg, MD, MS

Presidential Task Force on Patient Safety in the Office Setting (2008–2009)

Ty B. Erickson, MD
Elizabeth A. Buys, MD
Mark S. DeFrancesco, MD
Joseph C. Gambone, DO, MPH
Paul A. Gluck, MD
Douglas H. Kirkpatrick, MD
Sandra Koch, MD

Hector Vila Jr, MD
  (American Society of
  Anesthesiologists)
Patrice M. Weiss, MD
Sue Woodson, CNM, MSN
  (Association of Women's Health,
  Obstetric and Neonatal Nurses)

Staff

Hal C. Lawrence III, MD, *Vice President, Division of Practice Activities*
Sean M. Currigan, MPH, *Director, Patient Safety and Quality Improvement*
Pamela K. Scarrow, CPHQ, *Manager, Patient Safety and Quality Improvement*
Sara Kline, JD, *Deputy General Counsel*

The clinical information contained herein is based on a variety of publications of the American College of Obstetricians and Gynecologists, which should not be construed as an exclusive course of treatment or procedure to be followed. The clinical information contained in this manual is neither comprehensive in scope nor exhaustive in detail but rather is designed to provide general illustrations. The committee encourages the use of this manual as a resource in developing local criteria.

Library of Congress Catalogong-in-Publication Data

Quality and safety in women's health care / American College of Obstetricians and Gynecologists, Women's Health Care Physicians ; [Committee on Patient Safety and Quality Improvement]. — 2nd ed.
    p. ; cm.
Rev. ed. of: Quality improvement in women's health care. c2000.
Includes bibliographic references and index.
ISBN 978-1-934946-93-0 (alk. paper)
        1. Gynecology—Quality control. 2. Obstetrics—Quality control. 3. Gynecology—United States—Quality control. 4. Obstetrics—United States—Quality control. I. American College of Obstetricians and Gynecologists. Committee on Patient Safety and Quality Improvement. II. Quality improvement in women's health care.
        [DNLM: 1. Obstetrics—standards—United States—Guideline. 2. Gynecology—standards—United States—Guideline. 3. Quality Assurance, Health Care—methods—United States—Guideline. 4. Women's Health—United States—Guideline. WQ 100 Q105 2010]
RG103.4.Q354 2010
618.068'5—dc22
                2009045773

Copyright 2010 by the American College of Obstetricians and Gynecologists. All rights reserved. Printed in the United States of America. No part of this publication may be reproduced, stored in a retrieval system, posted on the Internet, or transmitted in any form by any means, electronic, mechanical, photocopied, recorded, or otherwise, without the prior written permission of the publisher. Requests for photocopies should be directed to the Copyright Clearance Center, 222 Rosewood Drive, Danvers, MA 01923.

The American College of Obstetricians and Gynecologists
409 12th Street, SW
PO Box 96920
Washington, DC 20090-6920
www.acog.org

12345/43210

CONTENTS

Preface   vii

Part 1.   Background   1

Part 2.   Quality Improvement and Patient Safety in the Inpatient Setting   7

Leadership   7

  Responsibilities of the Chair of a Department of
      Obstetrics and Gynecology—Nonacademic Setting   8

  Responsibilities of the Chair of a Department of
      Obstetrics and Gynecology—Academic Setting   10

  Credentialing and Privileging   11

Development of a Departmental Quality Improvement Program   12

  Quality Improvement Projects   12

  Creating Teams   12

Basic Approach to Quality Improvement   13

  Clinical Pathways   13

  Standards, Guidelines, and Criteria   14

Measurement   15

  Quality Indicators   15

  Performance Measures   17

  Data for Performance Measurement   18

Continuous Monitoring   19

  Peer Review Process   19

  Screening Medical Records   19

  Medical Record Review   20

Addressing Quality of Care Concerns   21

Physician Involvement and Engagement   23

  Patient Safety Leadership WalkRounds   23

  Safety Briefings   23

Process Improvement Teams   24

Physician Champions   24

System Improvement   24

Changing Physician Behaviors   24

Clinical Protocols   25

Perinatal Safety Programs   25

Department Meetings   25

Elements of a Patient Safety Program in the Inpatient Setting   27

Safety Attitudes Questionnaire   27

Assessment of Current Issues   28

Improving Patient Safety Through Teamwork   29

Patient Safety in the Surgical Environment   32

Medication Safety in the Inpatient Setting   33

Hand Hygiene   35

Use of Abbreviations   36

Disclosure of Adverse Events   37

Part 3.   Assessing Clinical Competence   43

Granting Privileges   43

Obstetric Privileges   44

Gynecologic Privileges   45

Credentialing for Family Physicians   47

Requests for New Privileges   48

New Equipment and Technology   48

After a Period of Inactivity   48

Part 4.   Quality Improvement and Patient Safety in the Outpatient Setting   51

Challenges of Developing a Performance Measurement System   52

Peer Review   52

Maintenance of Certification   53

Maintenance of Certification from the American Board of Obstetrics
    and Gynecology   53

Methods for Maintenance of Certification   53

Elements of a Patient Safety Program in the Outpatient Setting   54

Communication and Patient Health Literacy   54

Partnering with Patients   55

Medication Safety   56

Tracking and Reminder Systems   56

Part 5.   Tools   59

Data Analysis Tools   59

Run Chart   59

Control Chart   61

Histogram   61
Cause and Effect Diagram   62
Pareto Chart   62
Quality Measurement Tools   63
Plan–Do–Study–Act   63
Six Sigma and Lean   64
Failure Mode and Effects Analysis   65
Root Cause Analysis   67

Appendixes

A. Glossary   71
B. Voluntary Review of Quality of Care Program Overview   77
C. Measurement Resources   79
D. National Organizations Involved in Performance Measurement   80
E. World Health Organization Surgical Safety Checklist   88
F. Sample Application for Privileges: Department of
   Obstetrics and Gynecology   89
G. Report of the Presidential Task Force on Patient Safety
   in the Office Setting   91

Index

Index   109

PREFACE

The American College of Obstetricians and Gynecologists (the College) is devoted to serving as a strong advocate for quality health care for women and maintaining the highest standards of clinical practice and continuing education for its members. In 2000, the College published *Quality Improvement in Women's Health Care*, which joined a long line of publications developed by the College to inform and assist Fellows who participate in peer review and quality improvement activities. This revision, *Quality and Safety in Women's Health Care*, Second Edition, is intended to serve as a primer for obstetricians and gynecologists starting or managing quality improvement programs within their hospital departments or ambulatory practices by focusing on the following areas:

- Quality and safety in the inpatient setting
- Clinical competence
- Quality and safety in the outpatient setting
- Data analysis tools

The manual is presented in five parts. Part 1 provides background information on the evolution of health care quality improvement efforts. Part 2 provides an overview of quality and safety in the inpatient setting, including quality measurement, disclosure of adverse events, hospital leadership roles in community hospitals and residency programs, and patient safety initiatives. Some information may be adapted for use in the ambulatory setting. Part 3 addresses the issues of assessing clinical competence, one of the key elements of any quality improvement program and certainly a major responsibility for chairpersons of obstetrics and gynecology departments. Part 4 addresses quality and patient safety issues in the outpatient setting. Part 5 covers tools that can be used to analyze data or study management issues. Provided in the appendixes are resources that include the 2009 Report of the Presidential Task Force on Patient Safety in the Office Setting and the World Health Organization's Surgical Safety Checklist.

It is hoped that this publication will complement the guidelines documents, Practice Bulletins, and Committee Opinions from the College and jointly serve as the foundation for continuous quality improvement and evidence-based best practices in obstetrics and gynecology.

Hal C. Lawrence III, MD, FACOG
Vice President, Division of Practice Activities
The American College of Obstetricians and Gynecologists

PART 1

Background

The quest for quality in health care can be traced as early as ancient Greece when Hippocrates asked health practitioners to *Primum, no nocere* or "First, do no harm." In 1914, Ernest Amory Codman, MD, a modern proponent of health care quality improvement, stated that "hospitals, if they wish to be sure of improvement, must find out what their results are." He believed that hospitals "must welcome publicity not only for their successes but for their errors so that the public may give them their help when it is needed" (1). Today, the pursuit of continuous quality improvement through data collection, reporting, and application in quality improvement programs remains an issue that is of utmost importance to all stakeholders in the field of health care.

In 1951, the creation of the Joint Commission on Accreditation of Healthcare Organizations (now known as the Joint Commission) established a standardized process for quality assurance. The traditional quality assurance model focused primarily on evaluating single untoward events and individual physician substandard performance rather than identifying and correcting process and system failures. This model essentially identified outliers and, as such, was only able to address the small proportion of poorly performing health care providers or bad outcomes that fell outside an acceptable threshold. Consequently, there was no structured mechanism for improving the overall quality of care provided by the large majority of health care providers or outcomes that fell within the acceptable threshold (2).

Quality is defined, measured, and evaluated in a number of different ways and from multiple perspectives. In the 1960s, Avedis Donabedian, MD, developed a seminal model for studying the quality of health care by identifying three distinct areas of focus through which to evaluate health care quality: 1) structure, 2) process, and 3) outcome (3). Using this model to help identify and measure various aspects of quality, a great deal has been learned that can be applied to improve the quality of health care. Most quality measurement information is derived from data collected in hospitals or large health care systems and, as a result, quality assessment

efforts at the health care provider level or in the area of outpatient care have lagged behind those at the facility level (4).

In Donabedian's model, measures of structure evaluate the resources associated with the provision of care and the role these resources play in quality (eg, factors such as staffing, equipment, and space). Process measures analyze the practice activities that make up care delivery; data can be collected through direct observation of patient care or review of the medical record. Outcomes measures emphasize the end results of care by the health care provider or facility. These data are captured through a variety of sources, such as medical records, administrative and insurance data, and vital statistics records. Essentially, Donabedian's theory suggests that good structure contributes to the likelihood of good process, and good process increases the likelihood of a good outcome.

In recent years, the focus of quality improvement efforts has shifted from a punitive approach to an educational one. Ideally, the quality improvement process should provide useful information to improve the quality of care by all health care providers, at all levels of care. To that end, the ongoing monitoring and evaluation of clinical patient care can be conceived as a process that takes place along a continuum, as depicted in Figure 1-1.

The range of quality reflected in the practice of health care can be described by a bell-shaped curve extending from worst performance to best performance. The types of efforts designed to improve the quality of care can be applied at various points on this continuum. The first clinical improvement strategy is quality assurance (A), which is designed to identify, eliminate, and prevent substandard practice. An example of quality assurance occurs when a potential deficiency is identified through retrospective chart review but is later deemed as appropriate care through the peer review process. The second strategy is continuous improvement (B), which includes a range of activities designed to reduce variation in practice and move global performance toward best performance. One method of continuous clinical

1

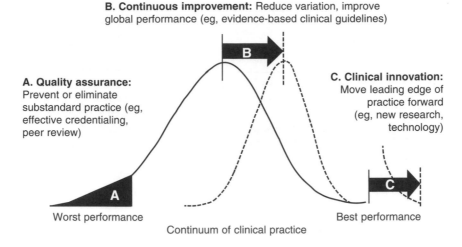

Fig. 1-1. Approaches to quality: clinical improvement strategies. (© 2003 ProMedica Health System, used with permission.)

improvement is the adoption of evidence-based clinical guidelines to encourage the reliable provision of care that meets best practice standards. The final strategy is clinical innovation (C), which is designed to move the leading edge of clinical practice forward through adoption of new innovation, technology, and research. An example of this is the adoption of liquid-based cytology technology and oncogenic human papillomavirus DNA testing for cervical cancer screening to improve the quality and predictive value of screening tests for cervical cancer. Collectively, these strategies work synergistically to optimize the probability of a successful outcome (5).

In the 1990s, major attention was directed toward health care quality with the publication of a report by the Institute of Medicine (IOM) entitled *Medicare: A Strategy for Quality Assurance*. This report defined quality of care as "the degree to which health services for individuals and populations increase the likelihood of desired health outcomes and are consistent with current professional qualities" (6).

In 2000, the IOM Committee on Quality of Health Care in America published *To Err is Human: Building a Safer Health System*. This report estimated that as many as 98,000 Americans die each year as a result of medical errors. The findings created a public furor that contributed to a widespread movement to improve the safety of health care. The report provided a number of specific recommendations for improving patient safety. Among them was the recommendation that "professional societies should make a visible commitment to patient safety by establishing a permanent committee dedicated to safety improvement" (7). To that end, in 2000, the College established a subcommittee on patient safety that would eventually become the Committee on Patient Safety and Quality Improvement.

In 2001, the same IOM committee published its second and final report, *Crossing the Quality Chasm: A New Health System for the 21st Century*, which called for fundamental changes in the U.S. health care system to close large gaps in the quality of care found at every level of the system (8). Although this report received less mainstream media attention than the first one, it has been heralded for the many significant recommendations that the IOM committee put forward and is regarded as a seminal document throughout the field of health care. Among the important contributions presented in the report, the committee identified six specific aims for health care quality improvement, stating the need for all health care to be safe, effective, patient-centered, timely, efficient, and equitable (8):

1. *Safe*—avoiding injuries to patients from the care that is intended to help.

2. *Effective*—providing services based on scientific knowledge to all who could benefit and refraining from providing services to those not likely to benefit (avoiding underuse and overuse).

3. *Patient-centered*—providing care that is respectful of and responsive to individual patient preferences, needs, and values and ensuring that patient values guide all clinical decisions.

4. *Timely*—reducing waits and sometimes harmful delays for both those who receive and those who give care.

5. *Efficient*—avoiding waste, in particular waste of equipment, supplies, ideas, and energy.

6. *Equitable*—providing care that does not vary in quality because of personal characteristics such as gender, ethnicity, geographic location, and socioeconomic status.

The IOM committee also proposed 10 rules for redesign of the 21st century health care system (8):

1. *Care is based on continuous healing relationships.* Patients should receive care whenever they need it and in many forms, not just face-to-face visits.

2. *Care is customized according to patient needs and values.* The system should be designed to meet the most common types of needs but should have the capability to respond to individual patient choices and preferences.

3. *The patient is the source of control.* Patients should be given the necessary information and opportunity to exercise the degree of control they choose over health care decisions that affect them.

4. *Knowledge is shared and information flows freely.* Patients should have unfettered access to their own medical information and to clinical knowledge.

5. *Decision making is evidence-based.* Patients should receive care based on the best available scientific knowledge.

6. *Safety is a system property.* Patients should be safe from injury caused by the care system.

7. *Transparency is necessary.* The system should make available to patients and their families information that enables them to make informed decisions when selecting a health plan, hospital, or clinical practice, or when choosing among alternative treatments.

8. *Needs are anticipated.* The system should anticipate patient needs, rather than simply react to events.

9. *Waste is continuously decreased.* The system should not waste resources or patient time.

10. *Cooperation among clinicians is a priority.* Clinicians and institutions should actively collaborate and communicate to ensure an appropriate exchange of information and coordination of care.

The release of these IOM reports greatly fortified the interest in systems approaches to patient safety, which could include the study of human factors as they relate to the commission of errors, but placed them within the context of a larger system of contributing factors. The IOM defined error as "the failure of a planned action to be completed as intended (ie, error of execution) or the use of a wrong plan to achieve an aim (ie, error of planning)" (7).

The work of James T. Reason, MD, a clinical psychologist and professor of psychology in the field of human error at the University of Manchester, has been widely embraced by the quality improvement community. According to Reason, the traditional approach to human error has focused solely on the person committing unsafe acts—errors and procedural violations—who he described as being at the "sharp end" (ie, personnel or parts of the health care system in direct contact with patients) of the collection of issues that ultimately culminate in the occurrence of an unintended outcome. Reason postulates that errors cannot be overcome simply by attempting to correct the human behavior in each case. Rather, he points out that humans are by nature fallible and errors are to be expected; therefore, he suggests implementing system protections that reduce unwanted variability and increase the reliability of care processes. His underlying message is that although the human condition cannot be changed, the conditions under which humans work can be changed (9).

Reason refers to the "Swiss cheese model of system accidents" to demonstrate how, when certain conditions align by chance, like holes in slices of Swiss cheese, the holes in multiple defenses, barriers, and safeguards may be penetrated by an accident trajectory (Fig. 1-2). To help explain how this may happen, consider the following example: A physician is called at 2 AM by a nurse to get orders on a patient who was just admitted. The nurse is fatigued, having worked a double shift, and is overwhelmed because she is also caring for seven other patients. It is obvious from the conversation that the patient needs antibiotics immediately, but the physician believes she does not need to be seen until morning rounds. Without asking about the patient's allergies, the physician prescribes ampicillin for a patient who is allergic to penicillin. If the nurse had the patient's complete history, she would have alerted the physician to the allergy and the physician would have changed the order. This information was never obtained, however, and the nurse takes the order to the pharmacy. The staff in the pharmacy are swamped with new admissions, and an inexperienced pharmacy intern is working at the pharmacy window. Although no medication should be released until an allergy history is checked, this does not happen, and the ampicillin is sent back to the floor. The first nurse, still behind, turns to her colleague to hang the ampicillin. The second nurse assumes the allergy history was obtained and hangs the ampicillin, thus causing a serious allergic reaction.

This hypothetical example illustrates how almost any serious adverse event is caused by the alignment of a series of mishaps and system failures at different points leading up to the event, even though one could contend in this instance that the nurse who administered the wrong medication to a gravely allergic patient is the "one" who committed the error.

Physicians are socialized in medical school and residency to strive for error-free practice of medicine and to meet the expectation of perfection (10), and in this way, the delusion of infallibility is reinforced (11). Most

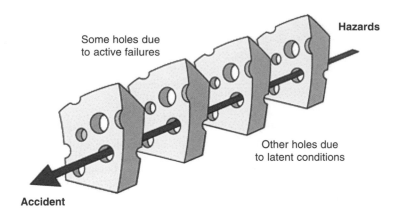

Successive layers of defenses

Fig. 1-2. Swiss Cheese Model. (Reproduced from British Medical Journal, Human error: models and management, Reason J, 320, 768–770, 2000 with permission from BMJ Publishing Group Ltd.)

errors in health care do not result in patient injury; however, because mistakes are inevitable, it becomes extremely important to develop systems approaches to reduce the risk of error and to implement processes to mitigate the impact of errors that may occur. Thus, the solution is twofold: 1) limiting the incidence of dangerous errors by building a better system of checks and balances and 2) creating systems that are better able to tolerate the occurrence of errors and lessen their damaging effects.

Lucian Leape, MD, a leader in the field of patient safety, draws upon the work of Rasmussen and Jensen on the nature of mental procedures that accompany the performance of skilled tasks to classify human performance into three basic types (11):

1. Skill-based—which is patterns of thought and action that are governed by stored patterns of preprogrammed instructions and largely unconscious

2. Rule-based—in which solutions to familiar problems are governed by stored rules of the "if X, then Y" variety

3. Knowledge-based—which is used for novel situations requiring conscious analytic processing and stored knowledge

According to Leape, as a person gains expertise in a given field, control of task performance in this area moves increasingly toward skill-based functioning because the actions become conditioned. During skill-based performance, however, many factors can divert the attention, thus increasing the likelihood of errors or slips. A variety of factors may contribute to the increased likelihood of committing an error, including physiologi-

cal factors (eg, fatigue), psychologic factors (eg, stress or preoccupation), and external or environmental factors (eg, noise and visual stimuli). Given the high prevalence of each of these types of contributing factors in the routine provision of medical care in general and obstetric care in particular, it is easy to see how prone to error physicians can be. This underscores the importance of protective systems that are put in place to help reduce the likelihood of error.

Conditions inherent in the practice of obstetrics, and to a lesser degree gynecology, can be compared with those that are present in fields that are operated by what are known as high reliability organizations (HROs) (see Appendix A). These include air traffic control systems, nuclear power plants, and naval aircraft carriers. A high reliability organization is one that has developed systems that enable it to avoid disastrous outcomes in an environment where there is a higher than average likelihood of errors or conditions that mean an error is likely to be catastrophic because of inherent risk factors or task complexity.

The success of HROs in averting catastrophic errors is related to some of the common features that they share (12):

- Preoccupation with failure—the acknowledgment of the high-risk, error-prone nature of an organization's activities and the determination to achieve consistently safe operations

- Commitment to resilience—the development of capacities to detect unexpected threats and contain them before they cause harm, or bounce back when they do

- Sensitivity to operations—an attentiveness to the issues facing workers at the front line

- A culture of safety—individuals feel comfortable drawing attention to potential hazards or actual failures without fear of censure from management

The aviation industry is the classic example of an HRO, routinely carrying out a complicated and risky enterprise that is relatively safe because of the highly reliable safety systems that are in place. The use of checklists, standardization of procedures, embedded redundancies, flattened hierarchy, and a confidential reporting system for adverse events all contribute to this safety system. The practice of medicine, however, varies widely for a number of reasons, and there is often resistance to standardization from health care providers. To reduce errors in medicine, efforts should be made to use the following mechanisms (11):

1. Reduce reliance on memory by using checklists, protocols, and computerized decision aids

2. Improve access to information at the site of use (eg, using electronic medical records)

3. Prevent opportunities for errors by using forcing functions wherever possible. Forcing functions are system designs based on a physical restraint that does not allow an error to be made, for example, a computer program that does not allow the incorrect dose of a medication to be entered

4. Increase standardization of high-risk procedures to increase the reliability of care quality

5. Provide targeted safety training, with greater emphasis on learning to think of errors primarily as the symptoms of system failures, to identify root causes, and to analyze failure modes and effects

The quality of health care has long been a topic of concern to those who provide care as well as those who receive it. Efforts to improve the quality of health care delivery, through attention to structure, process, and outcomes, and the application of new methodologies have evolved over time, with rapid acceleration in the past two decades.

References

1. Codman EA. A study in hospital efficiency as demonstrated by the case report of the first five years of a private hospital. Oakbrook Terrace (IL): Joint Commission on Accreditation of Healthcare Organizations; 1996.

2. Gaucher EJ, Coffey RJ. Integrating TQM and quality assurance. In: Total quality in healthcare: from theory to practice. San Francisco (CA): Jossey-Bass Publishers; 1993. p. 54–77.

3. Donabedian A. Evaluating the quality of medical care. Milbank Mem Fund Q 1966;44(suppl):166–206.

4. Starfield B. Primary care: balancing health needs, services, and technology. New York (NY): Oxford University Press; 1998.

5. Reiter RC, Yielding L, Gluck PA. Clinical performance improvement: assessing the quality and safety of women's health care. In: Hacker NF, Moore JG, and Gambone JC, editors. Essentials of obstetrics and gynecology. Philadelphia (PA): Elsevier Saunders; 2004. p. 46–54.

6. Institute of Medicine (US). Medicare: a strategy for quality assurance. Washington (DC): National Academy Press; 1990.

7. Institute of Medicine (US). To err is human: building a safer health system. Washington (DC): National Academy Press; 2000.

8. Institute of Medicine (US). Crossing the quality chasm: a new health system for the 21st century. Washington (DC): National Academies Press; 2001.

9. Reason J. Human error: models and management. BMJ 2000;320:768–70.

10. Hilfiker D. Facing our mistakes. N Engl J Med 1984;310:118–22.

11. Leape LL. Error in medicine. JAMA 1994;272:1851–7.

12. Agency for Healthcare Research and Quality. Patient safety network glossary. Available at: http://www.psnet.ahrq.gov/glossary.aspx. Retrieved June 8, 2009.

PART 2

Quality Improvement and Patient Safety in the Inpatient Setting

The Institute of Medicine (IOM) and other organizations have stressed the urgency of "transforming hospitals into places where each patient receives the best quality care, every single time" (1). In studies of progress in patient safety and quality, a recurring theme emerges: hospitals need to change systems to increase reliability. High reliability concepts apply not only to medicine but to many other industries, including commercial aviation, nuclear power plants, fire service, and law enforcement. Characteristics of high reliability organizations (HROs) have been identified as essential for any improvement initiative to succeed: preoccupation with failure, sensitivity to operations, commitment to resilience, and deference to expertise.

Preoccupation with failure refers to the attitude and action present when problems occur. Instead of regarding a near miss as evidence of an efficient system, such events should be regarded as a stimulus to analyze the event and build further safeguards to reduce the potential of harm to patients. Avoiding overly simple explanations of failure is essential to being able to understand the multifaceted reasons patients may be placed at risk. In addition, administrators and staff must constantly be aware of operational systems, such as equipment maintenance schedules or scheduled competency evaluations, and trained to recognize and respond efficiently to system abnormalities. The characteristics of commitment to resilience and deference to expertise are important for containing the unexpected when it occurs. High reliability organizations create a culture and systems that reduce risk and effectively respond when failures do occur. It is important to implement this sense of positive culture and teamwork in any successful quality improvement program.

Improving quality of care in a hospital department of obstetrics and gynecology requires numerous steps for process and systems improvement. This should always begin with strong leadership. One reason for this approach is to remove obstacles when necessary for making changes. More importantly, leaders can help energize performance improvement activities and promote a patient safety culture. Leadership should direct the use of standards, guidelines, and criteria for use in measuring performance. Utilizing these tools, care can be assessed and improvements can be made using various methods.

Leadership

Leadership has been defined as "a set of processes that creates organizations in the first place or adapts them to significantly changing circumstances" (2). Leaders define what the future should look like, align people with that vision, and inspire them to make it happen despite the obstacles (2). According to Parsons, Purdon, and Craig, authors of *Guide to Clinical Resource Management*, "the first and most important responsibility of a quality management department is to provide leadership for the development, implementation, and coordination of the organization's plan to improve organizational performance" (3). In hospitals, medical staff leadership roles and responsibilities vary depending on the organizational structure of the institution. Three institutional models are common (4):

1. Community hospitals with a voluntary medical staff

2. Hospitals with a closed medical staff (with or without salaried physicians)

3. Academic centers with medical staffs composed of a mixture of physicians employed by the medical school, hospital, or department, as well as physicians who have private practices or are voluntary, community-based physicians, or both

Regardless of the structure within a given hospital, responsive leadership in the department of obstetrics and gynecology, with support from the chief executive officer, the medical executive committee, and the governing board, is key to an effective obstetric–gynecologic quality improvement (QI) program and to the overall operation of the department.

Effective department leadership also is critical for spearheading and initiating QI activities. Leadership is the foundation for an effective program, providing support, funding, and resources. Strong leadership will be extremely helpful in soliciting buy-in from physicians and others within the obstetrics and gynecology department. Cooperation of departmental members will help minimize obstacles. The chair of the department ultimately is responsible for QI activities. (Additional information about the duties of the department chair can be found later in this chapter.) When physicians accept departmental leadership positions, their primary purpose is to establish an environment in which quality improvements can thrive.

A departmental QI committee may include the following members, with consideration given to the vice chair of the department serving as the committee chair:

- Representative physicians with varying levels of clinical experience (junior and senior staff) within the department
- Representative subspecialists, when available
- Certified nurse–midwives
- Registered nurses
- House staff member, when appropriate
- The department chair (ex officio)

The rules and regulations of the department should outline the responsibilities of the QI committee and provide information on committee size, term of office, and method of appointment. Policies for meetings should be established. Part of the role of this committee and the department chair is to create an atmosphere in which health care providers are able to raise quality issues in a confidential manner. Monthly meetings often are most productive and allow concurrent and retrospective case analysis.

The QI process should involve participation of all practitioners providing care at the hospital, group, and private practice levels. Participants in case reviews must be sensitive to potential conflicts of interest and scrupulously adhere to a consistent and unbiased process. When appropriate, physicians, including those from other specialties, physician assistants, certified nurse–midwives, nurse practitioners, registered nurses, and social workers may need to form a multidisciplinary task force to address specific issues that surface during the QI review process. At all times, confidentiality must be maintained. Minutes of previous meetings at which peer review activities are documented should be circulated only during the meetings themselves.

Responsibilities of the Chair of a Department of Obstetrics and Gynecology—Nonacademic Setting

One of the defining factors of leadership is the ability and the necessity to inspire. A department chair assumes the role of a leader. Some people are "born" or "natural" leaders and effectively inspire without really knowing or understanding the strategies or tactics of leadership. Others must apply a variety of tactics as leaders to effectively inspire and create passion and direction to an individual or group, consciously or subconsciously.

Leadership is not about changing a mindset, but about cultivating an environment that inspires and motivates a desire for change. Thus, the department chair must be an agent for change. Every individual has personal characteristics and environmental factors that contribute to his or her makeup. To lead, one should know the environment in which leadership is required and should understand why some members may react favorably to one situation while others may become frustrated, bewildered, or disillusioned within this same environment. The chair also must be motivated to lead and unify the department toward a common goal—safe and high-quality patient care.

The manner in which inspiration and direction is provided is called leadership style. There have been as many as 72 leadership styles and variations described. The U.S. Army Handbook describes three basic groups (5):

1. Authoritarian—The leader dictates how, what, when, and where the task is to be performed.
2. Participative—The leader includes one or more members of the team in the decision making process.
3. Delegative—The leader allows members of the team to make independent decisions.

In all three cases, the leader is still responsible for the decision. Good leaders will use all three styles as the situation, members of the department, and tasks dictate. Unsuccessful leaders tend to stick with one style.

In addition, to be an effective leader, the department chair must be willing to make a significant time commitment to this position. Besides being a leader and motivator, other roles may be required. Examples of these variable roles include being an advocate for patients and for physicians in addition to negotiator, arbitrator, enforcer, disciplinarian, counselor, innovator, visionary, influencer, planner, and evaluator. Planning, preparation, and carrying out the responsibilities of the position are essential.

As a corollary to the chair's time commitment, the hospital should be willing to provide a stipend for this leadership position. In recent decades, hospitals and physicians have experienced fundamental changes in reimbursement methods. Pressures on physicians' incomes and hospital revenues are constant and unrelenting. The gains made through hospital–physician collaboration and physician leadership should help foster the union between finances and clinical quality. Some of the responsibilities of the department chair include the following (6):

- Make recommendations to grant or withdraw privileges as mandated in the institution's bylaws
- Develop, institute, and oversee the patient safety and quality improvement programs for the department
- Provide a continuing education program for department members
- Establish and monitor policies, procedures, and protocols
- Serve as a voting representative of the department on the medical staff executive committee

The chair should become familiar with the bylaws, rules and regulations, and policies and procedures governing the medical staff. The chair will need to understand how governance works at the hospital as it relates to the department of obstetrics and gynecology. There also may be state laws, regulations from the Centers for Medicare and Medicaid Services, and Joint Commission requirements that apply to the department. Possessing knowledge and understanding of the hospital's and department's code of conduct policies will assist in dealing with uncooperative and disruptive physicians.

Equally so, the chair must recognize that not only is the department part of an organization, but that the department is a defined system within the organization. As such, the department, through the chair's leadership, must provide for a systemic culture of operational safety and quality. The chair should see to it that patient safety is the highest priority, that teamwork is emphasized, that communication is constant at all levels, and that guidelines for medications and procedures of high risk are developed and followed (7).

The chair in a community or nonteaching hospital must ensure that staff, faculty, administrators, and patients know that the care is, and will be, delivered in a safe and quality manner and that the patient safety culture involves them. Leadership support is necessary to facilitate the hospital's transition to a patient safety culture. Attitudes of the leadership and health care workers are a major part of making this change occur. Not only must the chair have the support of the hospital leadership, but the chair must have support of the health care workers and providers in order to succeed.

The way people work, and the systems in which they work, significantly affect what is achieved. Leadership is the critical element in a successful patient safety program. Leadership cannot be delegated and rests with the departmental chair.

Highly reliable organizations share several tenets. Patient safety is not a competition but results from collaboration. This collaboration includes standardization and protocols, nonpunitive approaches to medical errors,

transparency with patient safety as the root cause for achieving efficiency and effectiveness, and linkage of staff and physician behavior with outcomes. These attributes are key to creating a culture of safety. A successful chair will:

- Create a compelling safety vision
- Value and empower personnel
- Engage in patient safety efforts
- Lead by example
- Focus on system issues
- Continuously seek improvement

There are several attributes that contribute to a strong and well engaged leader. These include communication skills that enhance engagement, a systems focus, valuing and empowering employees, and continuously seeking improvement. Conversely, attributes of a weak leader include perceived lip service only, looking to assess blame ("Who made the mistake?"), allowing limited employee input, and accepting mediocrity.

In a qualitative and quantitative analysis through semistructured interviews and site visits to seven different hospitals, the authors of an analysis found that although many hospital leaders created a vision for safety, what distinguished strong leadership from weak leadership were the following factors (8):

- Extensive engagement of senior leaders
- Systems focus
- Valuing and empowering employees to act on behalf of patient safety
- Dissatisfaction with current safety performance

A chair who is a leader brings administrators, managers, and the medical staff together to promote improvement by establishing and demonstrating a commitment to the value of patient safety, providing adequate resources to build or maintain a culture of patient safety, and adhering to reliable, evidence-based practices.

Leaders can promote patient safety by adopting a number of action strategies as follows:

- Placing safety issues prominently on all meeting agendas
- Visiting with staff and asking about safety issues
- Assigning executives to safety performance improvement teams and reviewing outcomes regularly
- Including patient safety in all orientations or requiring separate patient safety orientations for staff
- Holding regularly scheduled briefings from staff working on key patient safety projects and asking how the leadership may be helpful in supporting this work

Responsibilities of the Chair of a Department of Obstetrics and Gynecology—Academic Setting

It is during residency that long-lasting attitudes and behaviors are ingrained regarding diagnosis, treatment, and interaction with patients and other health care providers. The department chair has a critical leadership role in this educational process.

Patient safety principles and practice should be part of didactic learning as well as the experiential learning in the context of residency in obstetrics and gynecology. To create the culture that is needed to improve the chances that patients will not be harmed by the health care they receive, both the structure and the language of education needs to change. Patient safety is a necessary component of graduate medical education to improve the quality of patient care and integrate patient safety concepts throughout the career of the obstetrician–gynecologist. This has the potential to improve care now and in the future by incorporating patient safety into residency training.

The challenge is to incorporate patient safety and quality improvement into resident education through the implementation of the Accreditation Council for Graduate Medical Education (ACGME) competencies (9):

- Patient care—Residents must be able to provide patient care that is compassionate, appropriate, and effective for the treatment of health problems and promotion of health.

- Medical knowledge—Residents must demonstrate knowledge about established and evolving biomedical, clinical, and cognitive (eg, epidemiological and social-behavioral) sciences and the application of this knowledge to patient care.

- Practice-based learning and improvement—Residents must be able to investigate and evaluate their patient care practices, appraise and assimilate scientific evidence, and improve their patient care practices.

- Interpersonal and communication skills—Residents must demonstrate interpersonal and communication skills that result in effective information exchange and teaming with patients, their patients' families, and professional associates.

- Professionalism—Residents must demonstrate a commitment to carrying out professional responsibilities, adherence to ethical principles, and sensitivity to a diverse patient population.

- Systems-based practice—Residents must demonstrate an awareness of and responsiveness to the larger context and system of health care and the ability to effectively call on system resources to provide care that is of optimal value.

This pairing of patient safety and quality improvement with the competencies can be divided into 1) didactic education and 2) experiential education. Examples and suggestions of methods to incorporate patient safety and quality improvement into the didactic education and experiential education follow. The associated ACGME competencies addressed by each are listed parenthetically (9).

1. Didactic Education

- Resident education should include didactic lectures specifically addressing patient safety (medical knowledge, practice-based learning and improvement, and systems-based practice).

- Morbidity and mortality (M&M) conferences should include explicit discussion of patient safety as well as the clinical discussion of patient care. When an adverse event is discussed during M&M, a discussion of the system deficiencies that contributed to the outcome should occur. Plans for a process and system improvement should be part of the M&M conference (practice-based learning and improvement and systems-based practice).

- Whenever possible, residents should be included as members of the hospital's departmental Quality Improvement and Patient Safety Committee. This will enable them to be educated in these processes and to be involved in the development of root cause analyses and other postevent evaluations, which should be multidisciplinary in nature (systems-based practice).

- Postevent evaluations (near misses, unanticipated events, and adverse events) are important parts of the educational process. Postevent evaluation includes a debriefing, which is a meeting of all personnel involved in these events irrespective of the outcome. Residents should participate in and may lead the debriefing session as appropriate (interpersonal and communication skills, professionalism, and patient care).

- Experience in using a structured tool to facilitate communication (eg, SBAR [Situation–Background–Assessment–Recommendation]) because communication, especially during handoffs, is an important part of residency education (interpersonal and communication skills and professionalism).

- Team training principles should be included in resident education. An example of team training resources is TeamSTEPPS (Team Strategies and Tools to Enhance Performance and Patient Safety) (practice-based learning and improvement, systems-based practice, interpersonal and communication skills, and professionalism). More information on TeamSTEPPS can be found in the section on "Teamwork" discussed later.

- Residency programs should develop resources that will assist residents and faculty advisors in dealing with their own guilt and emotions following their involvement in an adverse event that results in significant patient injury or death (professionalism). Disclosure of medical errors in the concept of the "Second Victim" will be addressed at the end of Part 2.

2. Experiential Education

- Residents need to be trained to include patients and families directly (patient-centered care) in patient care (patient care and interpersonal and communication skills) (10).

- Resident work-hour restrictions will result in more transitions in care and, therefore, increase the importance of well-executed handoffs for patient safety. Handoffs should be multidisciplinary (including residents) and structured using a standardized format (eg, tools, logistics) (interpersonal and communication skills).

- Recognizing that communication is a learned skill, residents must understand their facility's disclosure process and be encouraged to participate in the disclosure and discussion of adverse events with patients. Formal education in proper disclosure techniques should be considered in every residency program (systems-based practice).

- Residents need to experience and observe the four cornerstones of effective teamwork: 1) leadership, 2) situation monitoring, 3) mutual support, and 4) communication. Examples can be found in the curriculum of such programs as TeamSTEPPS (professionalism and interpersonal and communication skills).

Credentialing and Privileging

The department chair plays a significant role in the credentialing and privileging process. Specifically, this means the chair has the responsibility for recommending appointment, reappointment, and granting and overseeing competency of clinical privileges. Effective credentialing is the foundation of safe and high-quality health care. The initial appointment process has four main components:

1. Develop good policies, procedures, and criteria for appointment and reappointment—Credentialing starts with clear policies and procedures and minimum or threshold criteria that each medical staff applicant must meet.

2. Collect, verify, and authenticate all information—Gathering and summarizing information obtained is usually performed by the medical staff and office personnel. Source verification and documents required must be complete. No application should move to the next step until all information is present. The burden for completeness should be placed on the applicant.

3. Evaluate and recommend—This component requires the participation of the department chair, the credentials committee, and the medical executive committee. The application and supporting documentation are evaluated and references are reviewed and contacted. Evaluation for clinical privileges should occur during this step. The chair is responsible for developing the criteria for clinical privileges. The chair must be satisfied that the applicant meets the criteria of training and experience to perform the privileges requested.

4. Review, grant, or deny membership—Based on the recommendations of the department chair and the medical executive committee, the governing board of the hospital reviews the applicant's information and makes the final decision whether to grant or deny medical staff membership.

At initial appointment, a provisional period of a few months to one year is granted to observe first-hand the practice, judgment, and technical skills of the new member. Following this provisional period, full membership is granted but usually does not exceed 2 years. During the reappraisal period, all information and privilege requests are updated and the medical staff member may be reappointed. The review process is then repeated.

Specialized procedures that require additional training or experience beyond the predetermined criteria or core can be requested and granted separately. Privileges for performing a basic procedure using a different approach (eg, laparoscopically assisted vaginal hysterectomy), or new technology (eg, robotics) could be evaluated and granted in this way as well.

Recently, physicians who have dropped all or a portion of their practices and would like to reenter a full practice have become a challenge for department chairs and credentialing committees. Recredentialing and reprivileging these physicians require equally stringent policies and procedures as with the initial appointment. In particular, the department chair should determine whether formal reeducation, retraining, supervised experience, or use of simulation units is required before receiving privileges to perform a procedure. Because of the many reasons physicians decide to curtail practices and the various lengths of time involved, it seems likely that multiple approaches to reentry will be needed. Refer to Part 3 for additional information on physician reentry.

Development of a Departmental Quality Improvement Program

According to the Joint Commission, "performance improvement is the continuous study and adaptation of a health care organization's functions and processes to increase the probability of achieving desired outcomes and to better meet the needs of individuals and other users of services" (11).

Over the years, the focus of quality improvement efforts has shifted from a punitive approach to an educational one. The quality improvement process assists all health care providers at all levels of care. Ongoing monitoring and evaluation of clinical patient care should be implemented through a process known as continuous quality improvement. Continuous quality improvement is an approach to quality management that builds upon traditional quality assurance methods by emphasizing the organization and systems. It focuses on the "process" rather than the individual, recognizes both internal and external "customers," and promotes the need for objective data to analyze and improve processes.

The quality improvement process must focus on the total care delivered to the patient by an institution, thus involving outpatient care leading up to hospital admission and the patient's discharge and transition of care to outpatient facilities; care from physicians, midwives, nurses, and support staff; administration; and all components of care that contribute to a patient's hospital experience.

Quality Improvement Projects

Most obstetrician–gynecologists are dedicated to providing the best care possible for their patients. Quality improvement should be a continuous process to improve the health care of women while at the same time providing education to physicians. Deficiencies are more likely to result from lack of information or documentation than from improper management. Therefore, a strong departmental focus on education enhances quality of care and should correct most deficiencies that are identified. The QI committee should look at trends in care within the department and identify those areas that need improvement. When adverse outcomes increase, the source of this change should be identified. One should look to see if there is a clustering of events—the hour of the day, new instruments, new staff, new procedures, or an individual provider or other personnel. Current data can be compared through statistical analysis with previous years' data and with national statistics. This will target those areas that need improvement.

Once strong leadership has been established, the next step, based on the data collected, is to select a QI project of a process that is creating ongoing problems for others in the process (12). The key to project selection is to have data support a topic that is not too large in scope and can be solved in a reasonable amount of time. Data should provide information about the system, not individuals or departments. The scientific method can be used to define problems by stating questions, making a plan, formulating hypotheses, gathering data to test those hypotheses, drawing conclusions, and testing those conclusions. For a sample QI project, see Table 2-1.

A project is more likely to succeed if the issue occurs frequently and involves substantial cost, variation in practice, and easily available data. Other criteria for selecting good QI projects include the following:

- Choosing processes that managers and employees believe need to be improved
- Choosing processes that are clearly defined—those with clear starting and ending points
- Choosing processes that have short "cycle times," so that data are readily available and the effects of interventions are easier to study
- Avoiding working on processes for which change is currently planned or already underway

When the project is identified, "opportunity statements" should be prepared for use by the team. These statements should define problems and processes of manageable size but not mention causes or remedies. They should include measurable characteristics, if possible (13). At this point in the process, it is very important to obtain physician support; otherwise, the success of the project may be impeded. One of the best ways to involve physicians with quality improvement projects is to capitalize on their scientific training. Many physicians work well with data and tend to respond positively when given evidence supporting a project (14).

Creating Teams

For the QI project selected, a team should be chosen to include representatives from all affected services and areas to ensure that all the key stakeholders in the process are involved. By quantifying the problem and stratifying the data, one can invite the most appropriate people to join the team.

A manager or other leader who has partial or complete responsibility for the process being studied should be designated as the team leader. This person should be in a position to remove obstacles encountered by the team. Another key team member is a facilitator who can provide tools, techniques, and QI expertise to the team. The project leader, however, drives the project on a daily basis (15).

Effective teams should be multidisciplinary (including residents, nurses, and technicians) and should include members with three types of expertise (16):

1. System leadership—Someone with enough authority in the organization to institute change when it is suggested.

Table 2-1. Sample Quality Improvement Project: Improving Care for Maternity Patients

Topic	Samples Measures
A. Reducing cesarean rates, when appropriate, while maintaining or improving maternal and newborn outcomes	Total cesarean rates
	VBAC* rates
B. Improving patient experience of care throughout prenatal care and delivery, and after discharge	Primary cesarean rate
	Repeat cesarean rate
	Apgar scores
	Other maternal and neonatal morbidity and mortality measures
	Patient satisfaction survey scores:
	• Pain management
	• Knowledge of care of infant after discharge
	• Physicians' and nurses' answers to questions understood
	• Easy to find someone to talk to about concerns
	• Family and friends given enough information to help recovery
	• Told about danger signals to watch for at home
	Also: percentage of smokers who quit and don't relapse

*VBAC indicates vaginal birth after cesarean delivery.

2. Technical expertise—Someone who understands the process of care being improved.

3. Day-to-day leadership—Someone who works on a daily basis in the process being improved.

To reduce redundancy, which occurs frequently in team meetings, it is suggested that team meetings not exceed 90 minutes and be held no more than 1 day per week.

Basic Approach to Quality Improvement

Quality improvement efforts depend significantly on physician support, and physician leadership is crucial to the success of the quality movement (17, 18). Guidance papers and clinical practice examples for the development, implementation, and use of a QI effort in any health care practice are available (see Boxes 2-1, 2-2, and 2-3) (19–21). Before instituting QI measures, however, an understanding of the major components of a QI process and their complexities is necessary.

Clinical Pathways

Although precise definitions may vary, simply stated, clinical pathways are plans for the provision of clinical services that have expected time frames and resources targeted to specific diagnoses or procedures. Clinical pathways frequently are developed for high-volume, resource-intensive, and costly procedures. They are interdisciplinary, merging the medical and nursing plans of care with those of other disciplines, such as physical therapy, nutrition, and mental health. Clinical pathways are not standards of care, but rather serve as

reminders of interventions the health care team believes the average patient will most likely need. Deviations from a pathway are to be expected; however, rationale for the deviation must be documented in the medical record. Clinical pathways can be particularly useful as a framework for outcome management activities. A clinical pathway development process may include the following steps (22):

1. Define population

2. Identify pathway aim

3. Select work group

4. Identify measures of pathway success

5. Create a flowchart of the steps and outcomes of current process of care and treatment of this patient population

6. Identify areas of internal variability

    Compare to and analyze steps and outcomes of external practice(s)

7. Develop "best" practice (pathway of patient care)

8. Define specific changes to achieve optimal practice

9. Identify format

10. Define criteria for progression to achieve outcomes and identify potential variances

11. Define practice steps required to achieve identified outcomes

12. Validate or revise document with other process owners

13. Develop instructions for use

14. Develop implementation and an in-service plan for trial

15. Implement trial

16. Evaluate trial

17. Review document and instructions for use

18. Implement

19. Develop and implement maintenance and enhancement plan

The most difficult part is implementation because process improvements cannot be sustained without a planned effort to revisit. Refer to the "Plan–Do–Study–Act" section in Part 5 for additional information.

Standards, Guidelines, and Criteria

To measure and evaluate quality of care, it is helpful to compare it with some acceptable standard. Each department needs to develop basic guidelines about what should and should not be done in the diagnosis and management of obstetric and gynecologic conditions.

Much has been written about the development of practice guidelines, quality review criteria, and clinical protocols. The American College of Obstetricians and Gynecologists (the College) publishes guidelines as Practice Bulletins that are categorized according to the strength of the scientific evidence to support them. Through its Voluntary Review of Quality of Care (VRQC) program, the American Congress of Obstetricians and Gynecologists developed worksheets for use by nonphysician reviewers to aid in identifying practice variances that might indicate the need for further review, documentation, or justification. These worksheets may be accessed by visiting www.acog.org/goto/vrqc. Only peer review by qualified practitioners in the same discipline can determine whether such variances are appropriate. Additional information about the VRQC program can be found in Appendix B.

A department may develop its own screening tools or rely on tools developed by other organizations. Criteria pertaining to patient care should be selected, developed, and adapted by experts in the particular clinical area. Once drafted, these documents should be reviewed and approved by members of the department. This process will greatly improve compliance and acceptance of the criteria during implementation. Periodically, these criteria should be reviewed and either revised, reaffirmed, or withdrawn.

Regardless of the tools used, buy-in must be obtained from the leadership (administrators, physicians, and nurses) before development and implementation of these tools can be successful. The following suggestions may be useful in gaining physician acceptance of practice guidelines (23):

1. Identify guidelines that address areas of clinical importance to physicians

2. Establish guideline credibility

Box 2-1. Planning Data Collection and Management

- Write down the most important questions to be answered.
- Clearly define the aim of the improvement project.
- Determine what measures would support this aim.
- Design dummy data displays that will be used to answer the questions and fill them in with made up numbers. Does the data make sense when it is displayed this way?
- Make a list of the variables (components of information) that must be collected in order to fill in the dummy data displays.
- Write down the conceptual and operational definitions for each variable to ensure measurements are being taken the same way, the same things are being measured, and all agree on what those "things" are exactly.
- Write a simple protocol and follow it.

Nelson EC, Splaine ME, Batalden PB, Plume SK. Building measurement and data collection into medical practice. Ann Intern Med 1998;128:460–6.

Box 2-2. Data Collection and Measurement Checklist

- Make sure the intended use and analysis of the data are clear to everyone.
- Check that the methods of organizing, displaying, and summarizing data will provide the needed information to study what is of interest.
- Have clear definitions of how observations will be translated into measurements or evaluations.
- Be sure the method(s) of data collection will result in the acquisition of the needed information.
- Make sure the measurement methods are clear and simple, and that they minimize on-the-spot decision making or interpretation.
- Have a plan for recording other potentially important information that is auxiliary to the primary project.
- Verify that the measurement and data collection systems are embedded into daily routines and can be done in a timely fashion.
- Develop a measurement team that is trained to make the measurements and record the data; have an appointed leader of the team.
- Perform a small pilot study of the definitions, methods of measurement, data recording, and training.
- Seek "buy-in" from everyone who will be affected by the project or process by explaining the purpose of collecting the data and its potential use for improving quality of care.

Nelson EC, Splaine ME, Batalden PB, Plume SK. Building measurement and data collection into medical practice. Ann Intern Med 1998;128:460–6.

Box 2-3. Pros and Cons of Using Quality Indicators

Quality indicators can:

- Allow comparisons to be made between practices over time or against gold standards. These comparisons can stimulate and motivate change.

- Facilitate an objective evaluation of a quality improvement initiative.

- Be used to ensure accountability and identify unacceptable performance.

- Stimulate informed debate about quality of care and level of resources.

- Focus attention on the quality of information in general practice.

- Help target resources to areas of greatest need.

- Be quicker and cheaper tools for quality assessment than other tools (eg, peer review).

- Guide and inform for purchasing decisions and planning of service agreements.

Quality indicators may:

- Encourage a fragmented approach to a holistic and integrated discipline.

- Assess only easily measurable aspects of care and fail to encompass the more subjective aspects of general practice.

- Be based on dubious quality data and information that is difficult to access.

- Be difficult to interpret—for example, apparent differences in care may be related more to random variation, case mix, or case severity, rather than to real differences in the quality of care.

- Be expensive and time consuming to produce—the cost-benefit ratio of measuring quality of care is largely unknown.

- Encourage a blame culture and discourage internal professional motivation.

- Lead organizations to focus on measured aspects of care to the detriment of other areas and to concentrate on the short-term rather than adopting a long-term strategic approach.

- Erode public trust and professional morale if deficiencies in the quality of care are highlighted.

- Encourage massaging or manipulation of the data by health professionals or organizations if the results of indicators are published.

Reproduced with the permission of the Royal College of General Practitioners. Pros and Cons of Using Quality Indicators: The Royal College of General Practitioners Policy Statement: *Quality Indicators in General Practice.* http://www.rcgp.org.uk/PDF/Corp_qualityindicators.pdf. Accessed May 18, 2009.

3. Customize guidelines with physician involvement

4. Break guidelines down into their simplest and most important components; focus on decision points

5. Target the audience to reach only those people necessary to put a guideline into practice

6. Enlist physician champions to promote new guidelines

7. Make it easy for physicians to follow guidelines

8. Allocate the resources necessary to support guideline recommendations

9. Make quality—not compliance—the basis for physician accountability

10. Measure improvement and share the data

11. Keep guidelines relevant by updating them

Measurement

The tools used to determine quality or efficiency of care are called by many different names such as rates, instruments, elements, standards, indicators, or measures. Albeit differences in definitions are nuanced depending on the audience, for this section, they will simply be referred to as indicators or measures.

Quality Indicators

The primary purpose of quality indicators is to stimulate discussion (and action if needed) around improving the care of and services for patients. Quality indicators are defined as (24):

> ... specific and measurable elements of practice that can be used to assess the quality of care. They are usually derived from retrospective reviews of medical records or routine information sources. Some authorities differentiate "quality" from "activity" or "performance" indicators. The important issue is that a good quality indicator should define care that is attributable and within the control of the person who is delivering the care.

It is important to note that indicators are not direct measures of quality; quality is multidimensional, and many different measurements must be made before it can be fully assessed (25). Quality indicators are best used as a means of improving a system of care, not judging performance or being used solely as a management tool.

Quality indicators may focus on structural elements, process components, or outcomes in the health care system or setting under study. Except for the most common outcomes, there are multiple technical and practical difficulties in assessing outcomes. As a result, quality is most often measured in the form of process indicators. It is important to note, however, that process indicators do not signify quality until their relationship to the desirable outcome is validated (26, 27). Process indicators are particularly helpful when quality improvement is the goal of the assessment process, short time frames for measurement are needed, or tools to adjust or stratify for patient factors are not available (28). Examples of process indicators include medication administration and patient and family education. Examples of outcome indicators are shown in Table 2-2.

The Agency for Healthcare Research and Quality (AHRQ) has six criteria to examine potential candidates for quality indicators (29):

1. Face validity—The quality indicator should have sound clinical or empirical rationale for its use and should measure an important aspect of quality that is subject to provider or health care system control.

2. Precision—The quality indicator should have relatively large variation among providers or areas not due to random variation or patient characteristics. Precision allows for the accurate assessment of the effect of chance on the measurements being taken.

3. Minimum bias—The indicator should not be affected by systematic differences in patient case mix, access or resource issues, or other confounders. If differences exist, adequate risk adjustment(s) should be possible.

4. Construct validity—The indicator should identify true quality of care issues.

5. Fosters real quality improvement—The indicator should yield real changes in quality and not be subject to forces that would tempt providers to improve their reported performance by avoiding difficult or complex cases, or by other responses that do not improve quality of care.

6. Application—The indicator should have a high potential for working well with other indicators or have been used in the past. Using multiple indicators together may provide a more complete picture of quality than use of a single indicator.

Evidence-based clinical indicators can be developed following a six-step system (30):

1. Identify the outcome of interest

2. Form a measurement team to provide an overview of existing evidence and practice

3. Choose quality indicator on the basis of research evidence

4. Determine the standard of quality being sought

5. Design a reliable and valid system of measurements that can be consistently applied

6. Conduct preliminary testing for reliability and validity

Several sources of benchmarks of quality indicators are available for individual health care providers or practices, such as Healthy People 2010, the National Committee for Quality Assurance Healthcare Effective-ness Data and Information Set, and the Agency for Healthcare Research and Quality National Healthcare Quality Report. Please see Appendixes C and D for a list of quality measurement resources.

Indicators may be monitors of sentinel events, such as maternal death; if so, every case should be reviewed, frequently on an expedited basis. Indicators may monitor specific rates, such as with excess blood loss. If the frequency of a rate-based indicator exceeds the departmental threshold or there are changes in frequency over time, an indepth review may be needed. Indicators may be positive and desirable, such as detection and treatment of chlamydia, or negative, such as an unplanned return to the operating room. The Institute of Medicine has identified performance characteristics that would lead to better achievement of improved health and functioning. As indicated in Part 1, the IOM has proposed six specific aims for improvement, indicating the need for all health care to be 1) safe, 2) effective, 3) patient-centered, 4) timely, 5) efficient, and 6) equitable (31).

Indicators should be clearly and specifically defined so that they can be benchmarked and the results can be compared with regional or national norms. Risk adjustment methods (eg, body mass index, comorbidities, diabetes, and hypertension) should be used when possible. Deviations from the norm can then be readily identified. Physician profiles also may be developed so that an individual's practice pattern for each indicator can be compared with department and national or regional benchmarks. Such profiles will form part of the database used to make decisions on granting or renewing clinical privileges and can be used to show improvement over time. Deviations from the norm do not necessarily indicate inappropriate care. Use of a clinical indicator may flag cases managed by a particular physician that, when peer reviewed, appear to show plausible reasons for the variations. However, continued monitoring over time (referred to as trending) may demonstrate that this physician has a much higher rate of variation than the department as a whole. Therefore, trending data may suggest a problem, such as surgical technique, that an individual case review does not identify. For additional information, refer to section "Run Chart" in Part 5.

Institutions may wish to define acceptable levels of care (ie, thresholds) for different indicators. A threshold is a data point that, when reached or crossed, signals an outlier that needs further investigation and evaluation. Using thresholds is a method for deciding when an issue should be addressed and where first to look for possible problems without requiring peer review of all records. The threshold level chosen as the standard for the institution should be supported by the best available clinical and QI literature. Information on local and national rates of complications may be obtained from the respective state health data organization, the National Center for Health Statistics, or AHRQ. Thresholds may need to

Table 2-2. Sample Clinical Indicators

Obstetric Clinical Indicators	Gynecologic Clinical Indicators
A. Maternal indicators	1. Unplanned readmission within 14 days
1. Maternal mortality	2. Admission after a return visit to the emergency room for the same problem
2. Elective delivery at less than 39 weeks	3. Cardiopulmonary arrest, resuscitated
3. Unplanned maternal readmission within 14 days	4. Occurrence of an infection not present on admission
4. Maternal cardiopulmonary arrest, resuscitated	5. Unplanned admission to special (intensive) care unit
5. In-hospital initiation of antibiotics 24 hours or more following term vaginal delivery	6. Unplanned return to operating room for surgery during the same admission
6. Unplanned removal, injury, or repair of organ during operative procedure	7. Ambulatory surgery patient admitted or retained for complication of surgery or anesthesia
7. Excessive maternal blood loss	8. Gynecologic surgery, except radical hysterectomy, cytoreductive surgery, or exenteration, using 2 or more units of blood, or postoperative hematocrit of less than 24% or hemoglobin of less than 8 g
a. Required transfusion	9. Unplanned removal, injury, or repair of organ during operative procedure
b. Postpartum anemia hematocrit less than 22%, hemoglobin less than 7 g (decline of antepartum hematocrit of 11% or hemoglobin decline of 3.5 g)	10. Initiation of antibiotics more than 24 hours after surgery
8. Maternal length of stay in excess of 1 day greater than the local standard after vaginal or cesarean delivery	11. Discrepancy between preoperative diagnosis and postoperative tissue report
9. Eclampsia	12. Removal of uterus weighing less than 280 g for leiomyomas
10. Delivery unattended by the "responsible" physician*	13. Removal of follicular cyst or corpus luteum of ovary
11. Unplanned postpartum return to delivery room or operating room for management	14. Hysterectomy performed on women younger than 30 years except for malignancy
12. Cesarean delivery for uncertain fetal status	15. Gynecologic death
13. Cesarean delivery for failure to progress	16. Appropriate use of deep vein thrombosis prophylaxis for gynecologic surgery
B. Neonatal indicators	
14. Deaths of infants weighing 500 g or more subcategorized by intrahospital neonatal deaths, total stillborn fetuses, and intrapartum stillborn fetuses	
15. Delivery of an infant at less than 32 weeks of gestation in an institution without a neonatal intensive care unit	
16. Transfer of a neonate to a neonatal intensive care unit in another institution	

*To be defined by each institution.

be changed as new technology evolves and treatments improve.

Collaboration of 15 institutions resulted in the development of standardized quality improvement tools, which hold promise for a nationally accepted set of quality indicators (32). Using national quality indicators from the College, the Joint Commission, the National Perinatal Information Center, AHRQ, and other sources, consensus conferences were held to develop national quality measures. An adverse outcome index was developed, as shown in Table 2-3, which measures the number of obstetric deliveries in an institution that are complicated by one or more of the identified adverse outcomes (33). The adverse outcome index is one of several quality monitoring tools currently available. Hospitals must consider all possible options, including local resources, in building the most appropriate QI indicators for their institution. Refer to Appendix C for additional resources.

Performance Measures

Performance measures are designed to guide physicians in their evaluation, reporting, and delivery of quality care to patients. Although they may measure different components of quality, they should ultimately be linked in a meaningful way to outcomes. Currently, the major obstacle to improving the quality of health care in the United States is the lack of a coherent and consistent system for assessing and reporting on the performance of the health care system (34). There is a lack of consensus on what national performance measures should contain and what areas they should target. What is clear, however, is that stakeholders want more information about how the health care system is performing.

The IOM report on performance measures, payment, and performance improvement noted that current performance measurement systems are limited because it

Table 2-3. Clinical Maternal Neonatal Measures and Assigned Weights

Index Measures	Weights
Maternal death	750
Intrapartum or neonatal death (more than 2,500 g)	400
Uterine rupture	100
Maternal admission to ICU	65
Birth trauma (Erb's palsy, vacuum or forceps injury)	60
Return to operating room or labor and delivery unit	40
Admission to NICU (more than 2,500 g for more than 24 h)	35
Apgar score less than 7 at 5 min	25
Blood transfusion	20
Third- or fourth-degree perineal tear	5

Abbreviations: ICU, intensive care unit; NICU, neonatal intensive care unit.
Nielson PE, Goldman MB, Mann S, Shapiro DE, Marcus RG, Pratt SD, et al. Effects of teamwork training on adverse outcomes and process of care in labor and delivery: a randomized controlled trial. Obstet Gynecol 2007;109:48–55.

is not always clear that the criteria being measured are truly or solely responsible for improvements that may be seen (34).

Data for Performance Measurement

There are three main sources of data for performance measurements: administrative claims and enrollment data, medical records (paper and electronic) and registries, and surveys. Administrative claims systems are not designed to be specific and reliable tools for quality measurement and reporting. Paper medical record abstraction of data is time-consuming and expensive and electronic medical records are in their infancy in regards to interoperability, standardization, and use. Surveys of patient perception of patient care is attributed to a specific practice because either the patient identified one of the providers as their primary care provider or computerized algorithms based on claims designate a practitioner as the primary care provider. Both of these approaches are subject to error.

Data Collection and Information Sharing

Data collection is important not only to formulate the problem statement, but also to support the team's belief that a planned change will result in improvement. As mentioned previously in "Quality Improvement Projects," initial data collection is key for problem identification. Data also are critical for demonstrating that changes will result in system improvement. This is particularly helpful because not all change results in improvement.

It may not be necessary to collect volumes of data before effecting change. For example, sampling can be used to demonstrate the change being tested. Another suggestion is to use both qualitative and quantitative data. Process and outcome measures also may be used

to help determine whether a change has led to improvement (16).

Types of Performance Measures

Performance measures include measures of the health care process (eg, hemoglobin A_{1C} testing for patients with diabetes), health outcomes (eg, neonatal mortality rates), perceptions of care (eg, patient satisfaction with physician interactions), and organizational structure and systems (eg, electronic order entry). Standardized performance measures have detailed specifications; they may require risk adjustment or stratification of results across key subgroups. A key element of any performance measurement system is ensuring that the data for performance measures are reported accurately.

Performance measures should be designed to be used as a guide for physicians in their evaluation, reporting, and delivery of quality care to patients. They should be linked in a meaningful way to outcomes, but they do not necessarily have to measure outcomes. Process measures or performance measures may have some fundamental advantages over outcomes measures (35):

- Reduce case mix bias—Performance measures use opportunity for error rather than the number of patients treated as the denominator.
- Avoid stigma—With performance measures, the message may be more likely to be perceived as "improve this," not "you're bad at that." For this reason, they are less likely to promote "gaming the system."
- Prompt wider action—Process measures encourage action at every level of the organization, not just a few individuals or the outliers.
- Evaluate delayed events—Process measures are more useful than outcome measures for evaluating events that may take longer to appear.

Process measurements can be precisely defined and are often very specific; hence, they are not usually subject to risk adjustment. They are ideal measures to include as performance measures but only if there is an evidence-based link to quality improvement. It is not practical to set the threshold for measurement at 100%—too many exclusion criteria would need to be incorporated and result in increased data burdens on health care providers—but levels may be based on aggregate national data.

In the 1970s and 1980s, when the use of peer review expanded, instances in which the process was used as a punitive or political tool found their way to the courts; in some instances, members of the peer review team were held liable for monetary damages. This sparked the passage of the Health Care Quality Improvement Act of 1986. This act resulted from concerns that physicians would hesitate to participate in peer review committees, which could lead to compromised quality in health care. The Health Care Quality Improvement Act established standards for hospital peer review committees; provided qualified immunity in the form of protection from monetary damages for those involved in peer review, provided due process has been followed; and created the National Practitioner Data Bank (a mandate that hospitals and other health care entities, including insurance carriers, report physicians who have been sanctioned or subject to specific disciplinary actions). The act further requires hospitals to request information from the National Practitioner Data Bank for all physicians who apply for or have been granted privileges at their institution, including at the time of reappraisal (36).

Continuous Monitoring

Current medical staff standards from the Joint Commission require hospitals to evaluate physicians on an ongoing basis, rather than just a periodic peer review. Current physicians must be evaluated as part of an "ongoing professional practice evaluation." The Joint Commission has left it up to each hospital to develop the process and determine which indicators to use. Some hospitals are developing systems that employ the six core competencies used to assess residents. Although these competencies—patient care, medical knowledge, interpersonal and communication skills, professionalism, practice-based learning and improvement, and systems-based practice—may be helpful, the Joint Commission is not requiring their use.

Another requirement, effective January 2008, requires hospitals to establish parameters that trigger a "focused professional practice evaluation" of a physician, such as a sentinel event, a near miss, complaints from staff or patients, or not meeting benchmarks during an ongoing evaluation process. A focused professional practice evaluation also is required for new physicians or current physicians requesting new privileges such as new urogynecologic procedures or use of the robotic technology (37).

Peer Review Process

In the United States, the traditional method of peer review continues to focus on quality assurance measures. Many institutions use peer review as a component of performance evaluations, with a focus on retrospective chart audits (38, 39). The problems with this approach include reviewer bias, subjective assessment guidelines, and low interrater reliability (40).

In light of these flaws, tools have been developed to enable peers to assess others' professional performance in a multitude of domains, including those not amenable to evaluation through a written or clinical examination (41–44). The validity of these tools as actual measures of quality is unclear (44–46).

In a review of the literature on existing instruments to assess one's peers, researchers found a limited amount of evidence; the search was not limited to English-only articles (47). Their review included instruments that had been specifically developed for physicians' use in assessing their peers, and any that were included were required to have some information regarding the methodology of their development or their validation using psychometric methods. At the conclusion of their literature evaluation, three instruments were included for review: the professional associate rating, the peer assessment questionnaire, and the peer review evaluation form (48–51). Information on planning data collection and management (Box 2-1), data collection and measurement checklist (Box 2-2), pros and cons of using quality indicators (Box 2-3), and challenges for doing performance measurement in small facilities (Box 2-4) may be useful in guiding performance improvement activities.

Screening Medical Records

Accurate and thorough collection of data allows identification of cases at variance with established standards and, ultimately, determination of the quality of care provided. Chart analysis following discharge seems to be the most accurate method of data retrieval. Although charts may be reviewed on a concurrent or a retrospective basis, retrospective chart review is more commonly used for screening medical records for quality review purposes. Using quality indicators or screening criteria, a trained data abstractor should screen all charts of patients discharged from the department of obstetrics and gynecology to identify cases that require further assessment by the department's QI committee. A member of the hospital QI department or department of medical records generally is responsible for the abstraction process.

The medical records department should screen all medical records for patients discharged from the department of obstetrics and gynecology for variance from established thresholds as soon after discharge as the basic information is complete. For obstetric patients, it is essential that the maternal and infant records be screened together if they are discharged on the same

---

Box 2-4. Challenges for Performance Measurement in Small Facilities

- Cost
- Lack of infrastructure
- Lack of health information technology
- Lack of support staff
- Increased burden of data collection

Landon BE, Normand SL. Performance measurement in the small office practice: challenges and potential solutions. Ann Intern Med 2008;148:353–7.

day. Fetal monitor records should be included as part of this process.

For efficiency, the abstractor should collect pertinent data daily. Collecting data on a regular basis ensures that the number of records will be manageable and that only a short time will be needed to complete the task. The abstractor must be familiar with medical records, medical terminology, and, ideally, the specialties of obstetrics and gynecology.

When data analysis shows that the care provided meets established criteria or that performance goals have been met, the satisfactory performance should be recorded and the monitoring and evaluation system should continue. These results should be communicated to the entire staff. Parameters to help achieve performance improvement goals should be recorded, shared with all personnel, and used to improve the standards of the department. Such positive feedback and reinforcement emphasizes the philosophy that the goal of the program is higher achievement and not punitive action.

If patients' records are flagged as outliers, the abstractor should indicate the reason for flagging the record. This information can be tracked for each physician for peer review, trending, and feedback. Any records identified as varying significantly from the threshold should be referred to the QI committee for further chart review. When the data for a month have been recorded, the data collection forms are given to the individual responsible for QI activity in the department. In some institutions, the data are entered into a computer, where they can be used to generate a variety of reports.

Either a manual system or a computer program may be used to document the results of this record review. Data reports can be generated more easily and more directly if a computer program is used, but such an aid is not essential.

Another QI process involves the acquisition of information and concerns from hospital sources outside the obstetrics and gynecology department. These sources include the nursing department and hospital committees such as those concerned with surgical review, infection control, use of blood and blood products, medication use, and patient satisfaction surveys. Reports from such sources may identify a problem that requires evaluation of the department as a whole or a focused review of an individual's practice.

Medical Record Review

A qualified reviewer should review any chart that has failed to meet established criteria. Chart review is an objective evaluation of the case as documented in the patient's medical record. The cases identified for review in a particular month should be divided equally among the committee members, with a primary reviewer assigned to each case. Cases may be referred to a generalist physician for review; however, if that review renders an adverse opinion, it should be referred to a subspecialist for review,

as appropriate. The physician reviewer is responsible for reviewing the chart and determining the adequacy of care according to published guidelines, institutional clinical protocols, practice bulletins, or other sources. Deviations from norms (ie, guidelines, protocols, and policy statements) may be acceptable variations or actually may be deficiencies. When deviations occur, the rationale should be documented in the medical record.

Care must be taken to ensure confidentiality in the review process. A copy of the hospital's confidentiality statement signed by the reviewer should be maintained. Although it may be ideal for cases not to be reviewed by direct competitors or by physicians in the same practice as the person being reviewed, this is not always practical. The possibility of bias should be considered in evaluating the results of such reviews. Any provider who may have a conflict of interest or has participated in the care of the individual should not participate in the evaluation process. It may be possible to hire an outside reviewer for politically charged cases or cases where there is insufficient internal expertise.

Problems also may be identified through one of the following mechanisms:

- Provider-raised issues—The QI committee must create an atmosphere that encourages all providers to refer cases of concern and ensure that all quality issues will be handled in a confidential manner.

- Clinical indicators (refer to Table 2-1 for clinical indicators)—Using *Current Procedural Terminology* (CPT) and *International Classification of Diseases, Ninth Revision, Clinical Modification* (ICD-9-CM) codes for the indicators may facilitate the selection process.

- Case referral—Referral of cases from sources outside the department (eg, risk management, patients or family members, other health facilities, insurance carriers, and ancillary services) and information referred from the state medical board or other regulatory agency can be useful for assessing other potential concerns related to quality of care.

The primary reviewer should prepare a summary of the case to be presented and discussed at the next QI committee meeting. A consensus of opinion by the committee regarding the case must then follow. Categories of decision on a chart review might include the following:

A. No deficiencies found—care appropriate. Morbidity occurred despite appropriate and timely therapy.

B. Opportunity for improvement
  1. Insufficient documentation of care
  2. Incomplete preoperative evaluation or prenatal care

3. Overuse, underuse, or misuse of care
   a. Attending physician
   b. House staff
4. System deficiencies
   a. Staffing
   b. Ancillary services (eg, purchasing, supplies)
   c. Other departments (eg, pathology, anesthesiology)
   d. Administration (eg, training, maintenance, performance evaluations, organizational goals, and credentialing)

It is necessary to maintain a record of all actions reviewed to identify trends that are collectively important, even though the care provided in individual cases may not have been judged to be substandard or to require corrective action. Both institutional and individual databases can thereby be developed. These data can then be compared with regional and national thresholds, when available, to determine the relative quality of care in the department.

Patterns identified by trending can reveal much about the appropriateness of care. Practice variations and deficiencies, including complications associated with them, become obvious when similar types of cases are reviewed over a period of time and across all health care providers. For example, insufficient justification for surgery becomes a valid measure of the appropriateness of care, especially when analysis identifies one physician performing a number of such procedures. If trending reveals a pattern within the department, such as a high postoperative infection rate, the department chair may initiate a program targeted to correct the problem.

The department also may wish to establish thresholds, defining levels of care for different indicators. Institutions should define acceptable quality by determining their own thresholds (ie, the acceptable rate of occurrence for rate-based indicators). Thresholds may be based on data from literature or on national averages when available. They also may be derived locally through the use of statistical control charts that document local experience. Thresholds may need to be changed as new technology evolves and treatments improve.

A well-designed and well-implemented QI program will prove effective in clearly identifying problems in care. Some acceptable variations are found during the peer review process and require no action. There is value in reviewing those variations with the entire staff, some of whom may not be familiar with the range of acceptable care.

Following the evaluation of charts from the outliers, those variations that represent inadequate judgment, skill, or performance should be classified as deficiencies in care. When a deficiency in care is identified, there is a problem that must be corrected. When the quality of care is acceptable but could be better, there is an opportunity for improvement. Figure 2-1 illustrates a sample chart review process.

Addressing Quality of Care Concerns

When data analysis reveals an area of concern, a specific problem, or an opportunity to improve care or performance, a plan should be formulated to address the situation. It is important to first check applicable hospital and medical staff bylaws to ensure that they will be followed. When deficiencies in care are found, the department chair or the person designated by the medical staff bylaws should investigate and take appropriate action. Such action may be department wide or directed toward one or more individuals. In the latter circumstance, the hospital's legal counsel should be consulted and involved in the process at an early stage to ensure compliance with the bylaws and applicable legal requirements. Corrective action usually can be handled within the department. However, specific problems that may require further investigation and corrective action should be handled as specified in the medical staff bylaws.

Performance profiles should be maintained by the QI committee. Once a practitioner's performance profile indicates that the standards of the department have not been met, corrective action may need to be instituted and documented. The severity of the problem will dictate the steps that need to be taken. The QI committee may meet with the practitioner to review concerns. The appropriate information to correct a perceived deficiency should be made available to the practitioner. The practitioner should be given educational materials concerning the particular problem that was identified. These materials may consist of protocols, current literature, or other related materials. Continued surveillance through record review may be all that is needed.

If the QI committee concludes that a medical record reflects care that is inappropriate or of unacceptable quality, the problem should be referred to the appropriate body and documented as specified in the medical staff bylaws. Applicable confidentiality provisions must be followed. A member of the QI committee should be present at any hospital executive committee meeting at which the case is reviewed to discuss the case and the reasons the care was deemed to be deficient.

Despite the best quality improvement efforts conducted by the department, there may be occasions when a physician outlier is identified whose quality of care is deficient and who is not willing or able to improve. These types of cases may require progressively restrictive steps of corrective action. There also may be cases where remedial steps have failed or have been refused, or where there is a pattern of inappropriate or substandard care necessitating more severe disciplinary action.

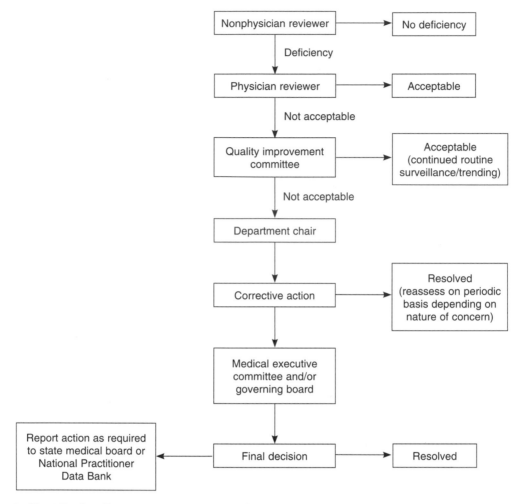

Fig. 2-1. Sample Chart Review Process.

The medical executive committee, the chair of the department, and the QI committee should determine which corrective steps should be taken. It should be emphasized that education is usually the initial response to most deviations from the acceptable care, whether the deviation occurs within the activity of the department as a whole or within the practice of an individual physician. The following options should be considered:

- Meeting with the individual to discuss the care rendered
- Individual counseling
- Remedial and focused education
- Surveillance of care
- External peer review
- Supervision of care
- Probation within the department
- Restriction of privileges
- Dismissal

Any recommendation that modifies a practitioner's privileges must be done in consultation with legal counsel and the hospital's governing board. The physician's confidential credentials file should document any discussion of the event that occurred, including the date, the individuals present, and the agreed-upon resolution. Final action on the department chair's recommendations for restriction of privileges is the ultimate responsibility of the hospital's governing board. Medical staff bylaws regarding due process should be followed during all stages of corrective actions. In addition, one must be aware of the reporting requirements of state medical boards and the federal National Practitioner Data Bank.

Ongoing review should occur to reassess the individual's quality of care. Once deficiencies have been corrected, removal of restrictions should be considered.

Special considerations need to be given to physicians who demonstrate disruptive behavior or show signs of impairment. Since disruptive behavior has the potential to negatively affect patient care, it is important to have a process in place for recognizing and dealing with this type of behavior. Approaches may include establishing a code of conduct and instituting a monitoring and reporting system. What is most important is having a system in place for resolving complaints by conducting investigations, speaking with the respective practitioner, as appropriate, and requiring formal counseling, if necessary. If the disruptive behavior continues or is egregious, disciplinary behavior may be necessary as outlined previously (52).

If a physician shows signs of impairment, intervention before professional performance is impaired is encouraged. Many hospitals have physician impairment committees. In addition, each state has specific laws establishing the reporting requirements to the respective licensing board. For more detailed information, refer to the College's publication, *Guidelines for Women's Health Care*.

Physician Involvement and Engagement

Action strategies to promote patient safety include regular safety meetings, staff involvement, executive involvement and review, patient safety in personnel orientations, and regular patient safety briefings.

A survey conducted by the American College of Physician Executives found that only one third of respondents were "very supportive" of patient safety projects (53). In trying to improve patient care, physicians encounter a number of obstacles with lack of resources, patient compliance, and clinician communication and culture among the top reasons identified.

To better engage physicians in patient safety, it is important to utilize physician champions and minimize disruptions during change. It may be useful to solicit help from a physician champion to help raise the level of awareness of and increase involvement in patient safety efforts. This applies to both academic centers and community hospitals.

Finally, to achieve the highest level of cooperation, it is important to minimize the level of disruption to practicing physicians in order to achieve their buy-in. The chair must be well in tune with physician schedules to minimize disruptions. The following techniques can be used for promoting patient safety:

- Patient Safety Leadership WalkRounds
- Safety Briefings
- Process Improvement Teams
- Physician Champions

Patient Safety Leadership WalkRounds

WalkRounds are conducted in patient care departments (such as the emergency department, operating rooms, and radiology), nursing units, the pharmacy, and laboratories. Senior leaders conduct weekly rounds to different areas of the hospital, joined by one to two nurses and other appropriate staff, and ask questions about adverse events or near misses and the possible factors that contribute to them. During these rounds, data are collected and aggregated by contributing factors and priority scores to highlight the root issues. The rounds provide an informal method for leaders to talk with frontline staff about safety issues in the organization and show support while addressing staff-reported errors. WalkRounds help achieve the following objectives (54):

- Increase awareness of patient safety issues by all
- Make safety a high priority for senior leadership
- Educate staff about patient safety
- Obtain and act on information elicited from staff about safety problems and issues

Discussions during the rounds and all analysis that occurs afterward must be protected peer review discussion for successful implementation. This process will help participants (including hospital leaders, clinicians, pharmacists, nurses in all phases of training, and medical students) to gain insights into patient safety as follows (54):

- Understand the roles of systems versus individual involvement in adverse incidents
- Understand good teamwork
- Understand effective communication
- Understand and apply concepts of how information is processed and how errors are made
- Develop strategies for understanding and preventing errors

Requirements of the rounds are knowledgeable, invested senior leadership and well-organized support structures. Participating in WalkRounds helps leadership witness the effects of budgetary decisions on actual operations. Seeing direct effects of actions, as opposed to discussion, can create a powerful inducement to change. WalkRounds are designed to correct and prevent medical errors. The work is integrated with other ongoing safety initiatives in order to support and complement the overall organizational effort and transform the safety culture.

WalkRounds serve to 1) visibly demonstrate patient safety as a high organizational priority and 2) allow leadership to learn from direct care staff and physicians about near misses, errors, and hazards that jeopardize patient safety.

Safety Briefings

Safety briefings are meetings that help increase staff awareness of patient safety issues, create an environment free of reprisal so that staff may freely share information without fear, and help promote the idea that the reporting of safety issues is part of the staff's daily work.

To reinforce a patient safety culture, leaders should treat error reporting as a welcomed act of providing information; share analysis of reports with all staff, not a select few; solicit ongoing input from everyone on how to adhere to or improve on processes; establish a patient safety committee with authority to review safety issues across the organization; and provide safety and quality improvement education in different ways to everyone.

Leadership support of patient safety efforts is crucial for success. Without the commitment of organizational leaders, the changes needed to improve patient safety will not be made. Consequently, senior leaders must focus on creating systems that support both quality and safety.

Process Improvement Teams

Improving patient safety should be a priority of health care leaders and managers. An emphasis on forming and empowering teams to deal with problems and opportunities for improvement is essential for cultivating an environment where patient safety is the primary focus. To lead patient safety improvements, medical leadership must give patient safety the attention and focus that is given to areas such as budgeting, utilization, and access.

This culture must not only address strong accountability, but it also must support clinicians in reporting errors freely out of genuine personal commitment and without fear of retribution. It is abundantly clear from the literature that without the visible support and commitment of leadership, this culture change will be fragmented and uncoordinated and will have only minor effects.

Physician Champions

No one person can singly create a culture of safety. Chairs must identify and recognize other physicians who share the passion for patient safety and leadership skills. These people are termed "physician champions" and can help promote successful implementation of any patient safety initiative. Physician champions take on leadership roles, usher change initiatives, and direct efforts that come down to one very important focus—the patient.

Physician champions may develop scorecards or sets of performance measures to improve patient safety. The physician champions then introduce and implement these scorecards as peers. Other initiatives may include medication reconciliation, adopting a new computer system or electronic medical records, patient care transfer issues between units, and communication between providers, including use of the Situation-Background-Assessment-Recommendation (SBAR) tool.

It is imperative that the chair not only identify physician champions but fully support and recognize them. The physician champion will feel empowered as a teacher, leader, and caregiver. These physician champi-

ons will then empower others to follow in the mission of a "culture of patient safety." The chair's ultimate goal is to apply high reliability concepts to the hospital through patient safety leadership WalkRounds, process improvement, patient safety committees, and the identification and utilization of physician champions.

Patient safety leaders are responsible for creating a safety vision, empowering personnel, engaging in patient safety efforts, leading by example, focusing on system issues, and, most importantly, constantly seeking improvement. To achieve these responsibilities in improving patient safety, a patient safety leader may:

- Establish the organizational value system
- Set strategic goals
- Align efforts to achieve these goals
- Provide resources for the creation, spread, and sustainability of effective systems
- Remove obstacles to improvements
- Require adherence to practices that will promote patient safety

A successful chair involves physicians, provides resources and expertise that allow physicians to help lead improvement efforts, includes people from multiple shifts and work units, and avoids having quality improvement staff design initiatives without input from operational staff.

System Improvement

When the data gathered indicate that change will lead to improvement, the changes then can be implemented in a system-wide manner. Educational processes can be instituted in one or more of the following ways.

Changing Physician Behavior

One primary responsibility of the department chair or leader within the medical staff is to facilitate changes in physician behavior. Physicians oppose change that they perceive will alter the delivery of quality patient care, threaten their livelihood, question their sense of competence, or limit their autonomy. Hence, techniques and projects that reduce income, challenge professional judgment, compromise patient care, or decrease decision-making authority are likely to fail. It is important for physicians to understand how proposed changes will be beneficial to themselves and their patients.

All change is invariably perceived by someone as a loss. Change can be stress provoking and can present an unknown future. People respond differently to fear of the unknown, and their behavior may be unpredictable. Every effort should be made to minimize or reduce the stress of change. Good communication is needed in these situations. Creating positive change requires effective communication. The following concepts may help in developing a communication strategy:

- Consistency—do not flip-flop or play favorites
- Clarity—present a concise message with a concise plan
- Courtesy—show respect, invite and encourage discussion and participation
- Honesty—be open and transparent
- Good communication—strive to talk so that people will want to listen, and listen so that people will want to talk

Change is made possible when the leader develops good interpersonal relationships, learns effective communication skills, becomes familiar with what is important to each member of the department, encourages patient-centered care, and employs evidence-based practices. Team development is one way to encourage change, particularly in interdisciplinary teams. Teams will involve more people, more ideas, and more energy. Teams tend to maximize a leader's effectiveness and provide multiple perspectives. Listed are eight steps for successful change initiatives (55):

1. Create a sense of urgency
2. Form a powerful guiding coalition
3. Create the change vision and strategy
4. Communicate the vision
5. Empower others to act on the vision
6. Plan for and create short-term wins
7. Consolidate improvements and keep the momentum for change moving
8. Incorporate the new approaches

Clinical Protocols

Experts suggest that substantial quality improvements can be achieved by eliminating unnecessary variation in treatment plans (56). The QI committee can develop a draft protocol addressing a particular issue with the entire staff amending it to meet their needs. Once the protocol has been finalized, staff should be reminded that they may deviate from the protocol as long as the record reflects awareness of the protocol and documents the rationale and reasoning for not following it.

Perinatal Safety Programs

Reviews of obstetric care, including those performed through the American College of Obstetricians and Gynecologists' VRQC program, have demonstrated recurring issues that present obstacles to patient safety. The mission of the VRQC program is to provide peer consultations to departments of obstetrics and gynecology, assess the quality of care provided, and suggest

possible alternative actions for improvement. This is accomplished by way of a site visit conducted by three board-certified, practicing obstetrician–gynecologists and a nurse with experience in obstetrics and gynecology, utilizing various quality assessment techniques, including an evaluation based on the College's guidelines. The VRQC program has found that lack of coherent, collaborative communication among members of the health care team is one of the most common obstacles to patient safety. Other examples include lack of documentation of clinical events; performing procedures (such as induction of labor) without clinical indications; failure to carefully confirm fetal maturity parameters before delivery by labor induction or elective cesarean delivery; and other individual and team issues. Several programs exist that serve to comprehensively improve the level of perinatal patient safety (57).

The *Idealized Design of Perinatal Care* is an Institute for Health Care Improvement project that presents components, based on reliability science principles, which are designed to create safer perinatal care. This project has demonstrated that poor documentation and failure of communication between medical personnel are responsible for many adverse events in obstetric care. The *Idealized Design* model recommends clinical processes that decrease the incidence of team communication problems, providing a common language for team members. In addition, the program introduces standardized clinical "bundles" or interventions for specific problem areas, such as elective induction (58).

Another program that offers processes to enhance perinatal patient safety is the MORE[OB] (Managing Obstetrical Risk Efficiently) program. This program involves extensive training of team members, promoting a culture that values communication, and advancing clinical knowledge (59).

Department Meetings

Regular departmental meetings can be used to educate practitioners about improvement of quality of care. This might be a good forum in which to discuss documentation errors, such as failure to include a treatment plan and to sign and date all notes in the record, as well as to discuss how to make a correction in the record. Regular meetings of the department also can be used to address specific clinical issues. These meetings would allow the team member to present a problem case anonymously, discuss the issues, and review the literature and the methods that have been used by others to resolve the problem. Discussion can center around which practice guidelines can be incorporated into the department protocol and how to implement those changes. This method of teaching reinforces the need to improve processes at a department level rather than address the problem on an individual basis.

Presentations also may review complicated cases or difficult situations that were handled appropriately. These cases serve to identify which methods and treatments work well and can be used as the basis for protocols and improvement of care.

For small hospitals where effective peer review may be difficult because of antitrust considerations, it may be helpful to develop a relationship with another hospital to conduct peer review. In some instances, it may be advisable to arrange for outside, independent peer review. In either case, it is important to remember that responsibility for peer review and quality improvement rests with the hospital medical staff and, ultimately, the governing board.

Conducting Meetings

As with leadership styles, there are also meeting management styles. The two most prominent styles are chairing and facilitating. In these two distinct styles, each has its strengths and proper usage.

Chairing is useful at the start of a meeting when previous minutes, standing reports, and statistics are shared. Chairing will typically use parliamentary procedures, such as *Robert's Rules of Order* or *Sturgis Standard Code of Parliamentary Procedure*. When chairing is used during the discussion portion of a meeting, the chair is usually not neutral and may influence decisions. This is a major drawback. It is not uncommon for the chairperson to make important and final decisions on some items. As a consequence, the chairperson is often seen as owning the item, or that the decision was predetermined. This will often stifle participation by other members.

Facilitating is designed to encourage full and equal participation of all members when decisions are to be made. Facilitators should be neutral and thus empower members. Facilitators rely on collaboration and consensus to reach decisions. When facilitation is used, the entire group feels it has ownership in the decision making process.

Good meeting management is most effective when both styles are combined. The meeting leader may use a chairperson approach to start the meeting and take care of the routine and information sharing portions of the agenda, and then switch to facilitation to get input and foster participation on items that require decisions and group ownership. Developing a meeting management style takes time. An example of a standard meeting agenda follows:

1. Call to order
2. Approval of minutes
3. Standing reports
   - Administration (Vice President, Performance Improvement; Chief Medical Officer)
   - Obstetric-nursing Director
   - Surgery-nursing Director
   - Subcommittees
4. Old business
5. New business
6. Adjournment

A defined meeting process minimizes divergence, allows for an orderly conduct of business, and provides a motivation for attendance. Using informatics for pre-meeting communication and knowledge sharing is helpful. Informatics can also be helpful in the use of data gathering to support decisions.

All members' responsibilities during the meeting should be clearly defined. It is important that someone is responsible for taking minutes and someone else keeps track of time and time restraints. All decisions and plans should be documented.

Some department chairs may choose to include peer review, mortality and morbidity, and quality and safety issues during department meetings. The size of the department and member participation will usually determine the feasibility of adding these topics to the discussion. Issues of confidentiality and privacy must also be considered. Separate subcommittee meetings of the department may be needed to address these issues.

There are four basics types of meetings. The appropriate type of meeting depends on the task to be accomplished.

1. Briefing—Used for rapid information exchange and clarification. The process is leader dominated and there is usually minimal discussion.

2. Negotiation—Used for settlement of an issue. All sides are usually equally represented and the leader is usually neutral. The goal is to seek areas of agreement.

3. Problem Solving—Used for defining the elements of a problem and finding the elements of a solution. The leader is actually a facilitator. This process uses such techniques as brainstorming, SWOT (Strength–Weakness–Opportunity–Threat) analysis, the nominal group technique, and others.

4. Parliamentary—Used to legitimate policy decisions and offers mechanisms to limit debate. Participation is usually representative. The leader may be dominant or the facilitator. Rules of order are established. This is the type of meeting that is used for most department meetings.

Suggestions for Effective Meetings

Making the most out of departmental meetings requires advanced planning and adherence to a set schedule. Consider associating meeting attendance with privileging by updating medical staff bylaws to require staff to attend a minimum percentage of meetings. Listed are practical tips for making meetings work:

- Before the meeting
  - Plan carefully: who, what, where, why, and how many
  - Prepare and send out agenda in advance
  - Arrive early and set up the room
- Start the meeting
  - Start on time
  - Have participants introduce themselves
  - State expectations for the meeting
  - Clearly define roles
  - Review, revise, and order the agenda
  - Set clear time limits
  - Review action items from the previous meeting
- During the meeting
  - Focus on each problem in the same way
  - Complete one item before moving to the next item
- At the end of the meeting
  - Establish action items: who, what, and when
  - Set the date and place of next meeting
  - Close the meeting concisely and positively
- After the meeting
  - Review and sign minutes
  - Follow up on action items
  - Begin to plan next meeting

Information Sharing

Based on discussions during department meetings, a number of mechanisms may be useful for disseminating information to the department as a whole. These include:

- Continuing Education Programs—Variances identified through the ongoing QI process can be used to determine topics for continuing education programs. These multidisciplinary programs may address topics such as laparoscopic complications and shoulder dystocia.
- Summary of Morbidity Statistics—Periodically, the QI committee can present statistics for the department and share this with the staff to show them how they, as a department and individually, are performing. This would allow staff to understand the importance of what they are doing and how the changes they have instituted affected the quality of care.
- Newsletters—This method can be used to keep staff informed about changes and new protocols. Reminders about clinical guidelines, trends in the department, and the need for documentation can be included regularly.
- Electronic Transmission of Information—Electronic mail and an intranet service may also be used as methods of communication to reinforce education and teaching. They allow new information to be disseminated quickly and efficiently. The staff can be informed rapidly about a newly identified problem, recall of drugs, and defective instruments.

Elements of a Patient Safety Program in the Inpatient Setting

Assessing the culture of safety within the inpatient setting should start by surveying staff about their perceptions and attitudes on patient safety. Armed with this information, leadership can then determine where the organization is and decide on necessary systems improvement. The core of this activity should focus on teamwork and communication. While working within a team structure, staff can make improvements to various aspects of patient safety, including medication safety, time-outs, hand hygiene, and documentation. But when errors occur, disclosure to patients and their families, with concern for the providers as well, will be important.

Safety Attitudes Questionnaire

As health care organizations strive to improve, more organizations are recognizing the importance of establishing a culture of safety. The safety culture of an organization is the product of individual and group values, attitudes, and behaviors that determine physician and institutional commitment to patient safety. A critical step for continuous improvement of this culture of safety is to measure it and examine trends over time. A number of different tools are available to aid institutions in assessing their current safety status, which may help in choosing goals for improvement.

Organizations with effective safety cultures share a constant commitment to safety as a highest priority. Patient safety should always trump productivity of the institution when these two variables are in conflict. One way to understand the values and attitudes of the entire organization is to survey all elements of the health care team, including physicians, nurses, hospital employees, administrators, hospital board members, and anyone who will affect the culture of safety. Including more members of the health care team in a survey leads to greater validity of the data and more useful data.

Once a safety survey has been selected, a hospital-wide campaign should be considered to promote participation. A letter to kick off the campaign from the chief of staff, hospital chief executive officer, chair of the hospital governing board, or other important hospital figures will help to achieve full participation. Campaign posters, e-mail reminders, and announcements at various committee and board meetings are just some of the potential techniques. While many surveys will be done on paper, there are additional benefits to doing an electronic, online survey. Participants should be guaranteed anonymity and confidentiality, which may be promoted by electronic surveys. Electronic surveys also would simplify, and likely make more accurate, the data collection, and would improve the ability to sort data by job descriptions, units, or other areas the institution would like to assess. Depending upon the size of the population being evaluated, there may be financial costs or possible savings to having an electronic survey.

There are several patient safety survey tools currently available, each with certain benefits or drawbacks. Initially, an evaluation of the number of survey items (usually in the 10–50 range), time required to complete the survey (should be less than 10 minutes to encourage full participation), and cost will help to make the decision about which survey tool would be most useful. Many of the surveys are available online for free or for a nominal fee.

Some institutions may find it valuable to utilize a questionnaire that has been validated through published research and for which comparative data is available from similar institutions. Other hospitals may prefer a study that can be easily customized to fit the needs of the specific institution and to address local needs and problems. Still others may choose a proprietary survey tool with no published data but for which the organization that owns the survey may have comparative data. Some dimensions that should be considered for assessment by the survey tool would include the following:

- Organizational values
- Institutional commitment to patient safety
- Communication strategies and weaknesses
- Behavioral attitudes
- Atmosphere of transparency (fear of shame and blame, ease of reporting adverse events, quality of peer review process)
- Organizational learning and commitment to continuous improvement
- Teamwork assessment
- Systems design
- Overall perception of patient safety

Listed are sources of some sample safety surveys:

- Agency for Healthcare Research and Quality. Hospital survey on patient safety culture. Rockville (MD): AHRQ; 2009. Available at www.ahrq.gov/qual/patientsafetyculture/hospsurvindex.htm. Retrieved June 9, 2009.

- Singer S, Meterko M, Baker L, Gaba D, Falwell A, Rosen A. Workforce perceptions of hospital safety culture: development and validation of the patient safety climate in healthcare organizations survey. Health Serv Res 2007;42:1999–2021.
- Just Culture Community. Outcome Engineering Behavioral Benchmark™ Survey. 2009. Available at http://www.justculture.org/benchmark/default.aspx. Retrieved June 9, 2009.
- Sexton JB, Helmreich RL, Neilands TB, Rowan K, Vella K, Boyden J, et al. The Safety Attitudes Questionnaire: psychometric properties, benchmarking data, and emerging research. BMC Health Serv Res 2006;6:44. Additional information about this tool may be found at http://www.uth.tmc.edu/schools/med/imed/patient_safety/questionnaires. Retrieved July 7, 2009.
- Press Ganey Associates. Safety culture: staff perspectives on American health care. Pulse Report 2009. South Bend (IN): Press Ganey; 2009. Available at http://www.pressganey.com/galleries/default-file/Safety_Culture_Pulse_Report_2009.pdf. Retrieved June 9, 2009.

Assessment of Current Issues

After the results of the safety attitudes questionnaire have been compiled, senior leadership, in conjunction with the governing board, must determine what steps may be appropriate to make necessary improvements. These steps may include a number of activities, such as the following:

- Implementation of educational efforts, such as team training, simulation, or drills
- Development or modification of policies and procedures to address error reporting
- Hiring of additional staff to address patient safety concerns due to inadequate staffing
- Using comparative data from the local and regional levels, if available, to guide improvement efforts

Another important activity is to assess patient satisfaction. Patient satisfaction can be defined as the outcome resulting from the patients filtering the experience through their unique perspectives and evaluating the extent to which the experience met their needs (60). One of the more popular patient satisfaction surveys is the Hospital Consumer Assessment of Healthcare Providers and Systems (HCAHPS), otherwise known as CAHPS Hospital Survey (61). Developed in 2002 by the Centers for Medicare and Medicaid Services (CMS) in partnership with AHRQ, HCAHPS is a standardized survey instrument and data collection methodology for measuring patients' perceptions of their hospital experience. The HCAHPS survey provides a mechanism for collecting and publicly reporting information about patients' experiences that allow for comparisons across hospitals locally, regionally, or nationally. The survey asks patients 27 questions about their hospital experience, including 18 items about key aspects of the hospital experience. Results from HCAHPS for 10 measures (6 summary measures, 2 individual items, and 2 global ratings) are reported on Hospital Compare (an online quality tool provided by Medicare) (62).

Together, the data from patient safety surveys (hospital employees) and patient satisfaction surveys (patients themselves) can provide valuable information to assist in proactive risk reduction efforts. This may be facilitated by establishing a multidisciplinary team, with involvement of senior leadership, to review the collected data and explore opportunities to improve processes or systems. Members of this team could include clinical analysts, nurse executives, the department chair, and representatives from risk management and performance improvement. Regular meetings should be held to review survey data, incident reports (if any), and informal reports. Collectively, these activities can help create a culture of safety. Box 2-5 lists tips for successfully creating such a culture.

Improving Patient Safety Through Teamwork

Some of the worst disasters, both inside and outside of medicine, can be directly attributed to lack of teamwork. According to AHRQ, despite abundant research identifying the skills needed for effective teamwork in medical settings and showing that teamwork will improve patient safety, the widespread implementation of teams across health care settings is generally lacking (63).

In commercial aviation, the largest loss of life in a single incident occurred March 27, 1977, when a KLM 747 jumbo jet collided with a Pan Am 747 jumbo jet on the runway in Tenerife, Canary Islands. In the subsequent investigation, several factors were found that contributed to this disaster. It was a foggy day with limited visibility. The KLM pilot was under pressure to take off to avoid exceeding his duty hour restriction, which would have necessitated canceling the flight and finding hotel accommodations for the passengers. There were some communication issues because of the accent of the air traffic controller. However, the most proximate cause of this accident was a lack of teamwork between the copilot and pilot in the KLM airplane. It was obvious from listening to the cockpit voice recorder that the copilot properly heard the communication from the control tower that the Pan Am airplane was still on the active runway. He did not clearly and assertively communicate this information to the captain. The result of this breakdown of team

---

Box 2-5. Tips to Create a Culture of Safety

- Educate staff to recognize that a culture of safety should not only provide safety to patients but should also include staff, visitors, and all individuals interacting with the organization.

- Engage physicians in the effort early to ensure ongoing involvement and buy-in to the culture of safety.

- Share lessons learned from root cause analyses with leaders as well as clinical staff.

- Develop and encourage use of informal means for communicating concerns, problems, and errors.

- Assign one to two clinical staff members to be on the receiving end of information about safety concerns. The staff must be credible and nonjudgmental; have good rapport with physician, nurses, and other clinical staff; and be comfortable asking questions in nonaccusatory ways.

- Take a proactive approach to errors. Annually select at least one high-risk process for proactive risk assessment.

- Study and learn from near misses. They reflect success in preventing harm and are opportunities to learn.

- Actively search for information in the professional literature about how to do things safely.

- Provide team training so that all staff members are aware of the organization's commitment to a culture of safety and know how to implement this culture.

- Encourage patient and family involvement in the care process, including the concept of a patient advocate.

- Share information about safety efforts with others at conferences, through published articles, and through informal communication.

© Joint Commission Resources: Patient Safety: Essentials for health care. (4th ed.) Oakbrook Terrace, IL: Joint Commission on Accreditation of Healthcare Organizations, 2006, 12. Reprinted with permission.

---

function between the pilot and the copilot was the avoidable death of 583 people—all the passengers and crew of two jumbo jets (64).

As a result of this incident and other similar avoidable tragedies, commercial aviation instituted a new way of training flight crews called Cockpit Resource Management, now known as Crew Resource Management (65). This approach fosters teamwork to prevent errors from happening and mitigates harm from errors that cannot be avoided.

In medicine, a disastrous outcome can be caused by a breakdown in team function. According to the Joint Commission, most adverse outcomes in medicine result from lack of team function, particularly breakdown in effective communication (66). This was especially true in their evaluation of perinatal injury and death, prompting publication of Sentinel Event Alert 30, "*Preventing*

Infant Death and Injury During Delivery" (67). The alert stated that,

> Since the majority of perinatal death and injury cases reported root causes related to problems with organizational culture and with communication among caregivers, it is recommended that organizations conduct team training in perinatal areas to teach staff to work together and communicate more effectively.

The solution was as obvious as the problem—better teamwork and communication prevents injuries.

Bridging the gap between team function in sports and team function in medicine was the lesson learned by Great Ormond Street Hospital from the Ferrari pit crew (68). The 18 individuals of the Ferrari pit crew, working as a team in a dangerous environment, are able to change four tires, refuel, clean the driver's visor, and give the driver a drink—all in 9 seconds. The managers of the Ferrari team were amazed to see the lack of teamwork when they consulted at Great Ormond Street Hospital. Subsequently, the hospital leadership went to Italy to learn team skills from the Ferrari race team that they are now applying to medical care to improve patient safety.

In evaluating the adoption of new technology, researchers examined the transition to minimally invasive cardiovascular surgery within Partners Health, an integrated health system (69). All groups had fairly good results, but there was one group that consistently achieved better results and another that was much less efficient than the average. The highest performing group had the most evidence of team behavior with preoperative briefing and debriefing. The lead surgeon flattened the hierarchy to create a team environment. In contrast, the worst performing group exhibited few team behaviors and the lead surgeon created a hierarchical atmosphere. Teamwork can make average people great; lack of teamwork can result in errors even by the most talented individuals.

Barriers to Team Implementation

Two issues are considered barriers to team implementation: 1) resistance to change and 2) the scope of work dilemma. Resistance to change is human nature. In the context of adopting team behaviors, the physician must change and become "leader of the team" rather than "captain of the ship." Other individuals, such as nurses, medical assistants, and secretaries, must learn to be more assertive as valued members of the clinical team. Mutual respect is critical.

Task-specific competencies are important, but in specific circumstances, as in the context of teams, individuals may safely perform a task outside of their scope of work. A physician may need to insert a catheter in preparation for an emergency cesarean delivery or a nurse may order an ultrasonogram for a patient with third trimester bleeding, absent a physician's order, based on protocol. Professional territorialism and egos, and not individual competencies, become the actual barrier (70).

Team Structure

In medicine, teams may be explicit, such as in an operating room, or implicit, such as in a medical office. Medical teams are dynamic, constantly forming and disbanding, focused on the care of one patient necessitated in part by the need for constant coverage. In the course of 1 day, an individual obstetrician–gynecologist may be involved with a group of nurses, technicians, and physicians evaluating a patient in the emergency department, while another group of individuals are caring for a patient in the labor and delivery room, and finally, assistants and administrative staff are seeing patients in the office or clinic.

A team includes at least two people who come together to accomplish a common task. The key characteristic that distinguishes teams from groups of people is task interdependency; individuals on the team cannot accomplish their goal by themselves (71). A surgeon cannot function in an operating room without an anesthesiologist, scrub nurse, circulating nurse, and surgical assistant. In the office setting, a physician cannot function without a medical assistant or nurse, as well as front desk and clerical support.

Many environments of clinical care, such as the emergency department, operating room, or labor and delivery unit, should ideally have an explicit multiteam system. In the office setting, team function is equally important but less explicit. In a multiteam system, there is a core team most directly responsible for the care of the patient. Core teams have, at a minimum, a physician and a nurse focused on the care of the individual patient. Several core teams work more or less independently in most clinical settings. In support of the core teams is the coordinating team, consisting of nurse managers, physicians, and administrative personnel. The coordinating team must be aware of the activities of all the core teams and of the overall needs for the unit. They assist the core teams by ensuring the proper allocation of human and material resources throughout the unit in response to changes in acuity and workflow. In some settings, most notably the labor and delivery unit, there is also the need for a contingency team. This predetermined group has an explicitly designated role for responding to unanticipated events, such as an emergency cesarean delivery.

Overall, having explicitly designated teams with clear delineation of their roles will improve provider satisfaction, prevent work overload, improve efficiency, and decrease errors in any setting (72).

Team Functions

The outcomes of adopting team functions are to improve team knowledge through a shared mental model, to improve team attitude through mutual trust, and to improve team performance with better accuracy, efficiency, and safety. There are four skills needed to achieve these team functions (73):

1. Leadership—In the context of the clinical team, a leader must manage resources, encourage team behaviors, and resolve team conflicts.

    —Resource management. Team leaders must be continually aware of available human, material, and facility resources in the face of changing workloads. Workloads may change dramatically due to increased number of patients or change in patient acuity, especially in an emergency department or labor and delivery unit. The leadership goal is efficient use of resources or mobilization of additional resources (ie, the contingency team) to prevent individual overload and fatigue.

    —Encourage team behavior. Leaders must periodically assemble the team to share information. This can take the form of a *briefing*, scheduled team meeting for routine planning; a *huddle*, to resolve unexpected problems; or a *debriefing*, after the event, to improve the process for similar cases in the future.

    —Resolve team conflicts. Even in the most cohesive teams, differences of opinion may result in conflicts between individual members. The team leader must help facilitate conflict resolution. If team members perceive problems that may jeopardize patient safety, they must bring it to the leader's attention. If the problem is not acknowledged or addressed, it must be verbalized a second time (two-challenge rule). If there is still no resolution, the team leader may use his or her best judgment to address the issue. Legitimate disagreements should be expressed respectfully, always from the patient's perspective. A valuable tool for conflict resolution is DESC (Describe the issue, Express concern, Suggest a plan of action, and reach Consensus). With the focus on the patient's well-being, not on the provider's ego, the right course of action will usually emerge.

2. Situation monitoring—Situation monitoring is a continuous process. The provider is actively and constantly evaluating the patient and the environment for any changes that might affect patient care. This leads to situation awareness, in which each individual appreciates the changes that might affect the team plans. By sharing this information with the other members of the team, the individual creates a shared mental model in which all members of the team understand the existing clinical and environmental conditions.

The team, as a group, can then adjust their goals and, as individuals, adjust their roles to achieve the best outcome for the patient.

3. Mutual support—The foundation for successful team function and especially for mutual support is mutual respect, an appreciation of the unique role and ability of each and every member of the team. If each team member is valued, there is no reluctance to either actively seek assistance because of workload or knowledge deficit or freely offer help when needed. Mutual support creates a collegial climate in which teamwork thrives. Mutual respect allows for constructive feedback, in which anyone on the team feels free to give, seek, or receive advice that will improve future team performance. To be effective, this feedback must be timely, respectful, specific, and directed toward improvement.

4. Communication—Communication failures are the most common root cause of sentinel events reported to the Joint Commission (74). Human factors, in general, and the complexity of medical care, specifically, contribute to communication errors. Team training strives to reduce these errors by implementing standardized communication tools, flattening the hierarchy so that individuals feel empowered to express their concerns, and developing a common critical language to clearly alert all providers to unsafe conditions (75).

Ideal communication must be clear, concise, and timely. There are several strategies that will improve the accuracy of information exchange.

1. Call out—Most useful during an emergency or rapidly changing situation, a call out is used to communicate critical information to the entire team. The message, addressed to the team, is spoken in a clear, loud voice. For example: *"We have a prolapsed cord. Place the patient in Trendelenburg, and prepare for a stat cesarean delivery."*

2. Check-back (closed loop communication)—The recipient of the communication repeats the order or instructions back to ensure that the information is understood.

3. SBAR (Situation–Background–Assessment–Recommendation)—A structured tool to efficiently communicate important information leading to specific recommendations. Below is an example of SBAR communication between a nurse in the postoperative unit and the covering physician.

    Situation—*"Mrs. Smith has a BP 80/50, P 120, and urine output of less than 20 mL per hour."*

    Background—*"She had a vaginal hysterectomy and repair for prolapse this morning with EBL of 500 mL."*

Assessment—*"I am concerned that she might be anemic."*

Recommendation—*"I would like to increase her IV rate, get a CBC, and type and cross her for 2 units packed cells."*

This communication clearly lays the groundwork for further discussion and decisions by the attending physician. Some institutions have added an extra "R" for "Response," indicating that the receiver acknowledges the information given. This reaffirms that the communication has been understood.

Implementation of Teams

Before any organization (hospital unit, clinic, or outpatient facility) embarks on team training, it is important to evaluate their current attitudes and willingness to accept change. The Agency for Healthcare Research and Quality has developed a survey that has been validated in the hospital and is easily adaptable to any patient care setting (76). By asking specific questions about patient safety attitudes, the employees realize that patient safety is an important concern of the medical leadership. In addition, the survey can be administered again after the team training, to assess the impact of that intervention and also identify remaining gaps requiring further attention. There is also a specific survey tool to assess the readiness of the organization to accept a team training curriculum (77).

TeamSTEPPS, an extensive team training curriculum, has been developed by the Department of Defense and is available without charge from AHRQ (73). This multimedia program includes an instructor's guide and resource kit; multimedia presentation material with slides, video, and interactive exercises; a spiral bound pocket guide; and posters.

Benefits of Teams

Well-functioning teams provide several benefits. Health care provider satisfaction improves dramatically in a collaborative team environment (78). With improved job satisfaction there is lower nurse turnover and absenteeism (79). Teams also help enhance clinical performance. Although studies in obstetrics are not conclusive, studies in emergency rooms and in primary care demonstrate improved outcomes once teams are implemented (78–80). Teams improve efficiency and thereby reduce costs through coordination of effort and decreased redundancies. Finally, teamwork eases the workload on physicians by delegating tasks to other members of the team (81).

Ideal team performance is directly related to clear leadership, well-defined goals, understanding of each individual's role, continual reinforcement of team skills, and institutional (clinical and administrative) support (70). Improved team function enhances patient safety,

benefitting the individual providers, the institution or medical office, and, ultimately, the patient.

Patient Safety in the Surgical Environment

The surgical suite presents the chance for medical errors. Adverse events in the operating suite occur relatively infrequently compared to other types of medical errors, although these problems often receive increased attention. The American College of Obstetricians and Gynecologists' Committee Opinion Number 328 states (82):

> Ensuring patient safety in the operating room begins before the patient enters the operative suite and includes attention to all applicable types of preventable medical errors (including, for example, medication errors) but surgical errors are unique to this environment.

Surgery at the wrong site is a totally preventable occurrence if proper attention is paid preoperatively and intraoperatively. The term "wrong site surgery" is used to refer to a surgical procedure performed on the wrong patient, wrong body part, wrong side of the body, or at the wrong level of the proper anatomic site. Although these types of errors are rarely reported in gynecologic or obstetric surgery, the potential remains for this type of error to occur. Many states now require that any wrong site surgery be immediately reported to their state medical board, which will allow for more accurate data on the type and incidence of these errors to become available in the near future.

In 2003, a Joint Commission position paper on this subject was released entitled "Universal Protocol for Preventing Wrong Site, Wrong Procedure, and Wrong Person Surgery" (83). The basis for the Universal Protocol includes three essential components: 1) a preoperative verification process with the entire health team, 2) unambiguous marking of the operative site, and 3) a final verification process in the operating room, usually referred to as a "time-out," prior to actually beginning the operative procedure. This process continues to be refined by individual institutions but now almost always includes the patient as an essential member of the team to ensure these errors do not occur (see Appendix E). Although the incidence of wrong site surgery has been reduced nationally, it has been disappointing to patient safety experts that such preventable adverse outcomes continue to occur with unfortunate frequency. Wrong site surgical errors have happened despite chart documentation of a properly done preoperative time-out procedure.

While individual culpability for wrong site surgical errors still exists, the key to preventing these errors requires proper systems engineering and process design to reduce the incidence. Although the primary surgeon has the ultimate responsibility when such an error occurs, it is essential that all team members (anesthesiologists, surgical assistants, scrub nurses, circulating nurses, and house staff) be involved in the Universal Protocol. According to the Joint Commission, "the risk of error may be reduced by involving the entire surgical team in the site verification process and encouraging any member of that team to point out a possible error without fear of ridicule or reprimand" (83). Several important factors have been associated with an increased risk of wrong site surgery:

- Multiple surgeons, particularly from different surgical specialties, involved in the case
- Multiple surgical procedures during the same operation
- Excessive time pressures to begin or complete the procedure
- Unusual patient physical characteristics such as morbid obesity or a physical deformity

When these associated risk factors are present, increased vigilance by all of the health team members is essential. Clear and unambiguous communication with all members of the operative team is needed to minimize these types of errors, especially during the preoperative verification process. Communication issues are frequently cited problems in patient safety, and these issues are even more important in the surgical arena.

Medication errors in the operating room present some unusual challenges because of the frequent use of verbal, rather than written, orders. Use of verbal orders will increase the likelihood of prescribing, administering, and monitoring errors in the operating suite. Communication issues are again paramount, especially between the surgical team and the anesthesiologist as well as the circulating nurse, to reduce medication mistakes. Because almost all medications are given intravenously or intramuscularly, the adverse effects of a dosage error may be heightened. The usual hospital systems in place to prevent medication errors often are circumvented in the operating room, and attention to a different process may be appropriate in this situation. The increased urgency and stress present also can lead to an increased likelihood of error. A full discussion of medication errors is found in the following section on "Medication Safety in the Inpatient Setting."

Teaching in the operating room also presents some unique challenges for patient safety. The expanding use of surgical simulators and virtual training techniques outside of the operating room helps to better prepare trainees before entering the operating suite. The ACGME written requirements clearly state the necessity for full supervision and assistance by qualified and experienced surgeons (84).

It is up to the clinical judgment of the supervising surgeon to allow increasing operative responsibilities for the trainee based on their experience, skill, and level of training. However, the safety of the patient is always more important than the teaching experience. Communication issues, critical for teaching in the operative suite, and the unique terminology (instrument names, surgical techniques, operative processes), must be understood and shared by all members of the team. A single communication error can lead to a grave patient injury even with the most vigilant supervision of a trainee. Outside distractions should be minimized in the operating room in general, but particular attention must be paid during a teaching session. Pagers, outside telephone calls, nursing floor questions, and other interruptions should be discouraged, if not prohibited, especially during the most critical steps in the operation.

Obstetric surgical procedures present a unique set of patient safety concerns, as attention must be paid to the welfare of both mother and fetus. Medications that are routinely used in gynecologic surgery may be contraindicated for obstetric procedures, and a thorough knowledge of potential fetal drug adverse effects is critical. Communication issues are increased as another team, the pediatric personnel, must be included in the planning and performance of the proper procedure. While wrong site surgery is a rare problem in obstetric surgery, attention must be paid to consent issues for additional procedures such as tubal ligation or management of ovarian masses.

Patients need to understand the risks and benefits of treatment, as well as alternatives to treatment, before a physician performs any procedure or initiates any treatment. The process of providing this information, answering questions, and obtaining and documenting the patient's consent is known as "informed consent." Informed consent is a discussion, not simply a form. For more information on informed consent, refer to the College's publication *Professional Liability and Risk Management*, Second Edition (2008).

Another model has been proposed, called "shared medical decision-making," which is the exchange of information and treatment preferences by the physician and the patient with agreement by both parties on the treatment to implement (85).

Medication Safety in the Inpatient Setting

Medication error is the largest single source of preventable adverse events in the inpatient setting. The adverse drug event (ADE) Prevention Study found that errors occurred at a rate of 6.5 ADEs per 100 admissions, and 28% were preventable (86). In 2007, the IOM report estimated that more than 1.5 million preventable ADEs occur in hospitals per year, or approximately one medication error per patient per day (87). In this report, more than 25% of inpatient medication errors were felt to be preventable. Current estimates of the annual cost of medication errors exceed $3.5 billion nationally. These estimates do not include costs related to lost earnings or pain and suffering, which often can accompany an ADE. There are many different possible sources of medication errors:

- Incorrect prescription writing (wrong prescription, illegible, use of improper abbreviations)
- Poor order communication
- Product labeling, packaging, and nomenclature
- Improper compounding, dispensing, and distribution
- Incorrect administration
- Lack of adequate monitoring
- Insufficient patient education
- Hospital system errors
- Drug–drug interactions
- Allergic reactions

It is important to understand that human errors can occur at any stage in the medication use process. Hospitals should, therefore, examine each step within their medication delivery systems to identify potential areas where errors can occur. Many errors are preventable with proper systems design. Research has shown that approximately 75% of all medication errors are due to ordering or administration problems. Recent technologies like computerized physician order entry (CPOE) and barcode and electronic medication administration records are two prevention strategies that may mitigate errors in these stages. The focus of medication safety should be on the "Five Rights of Medication Use":

1. Right Drug
2. Right Dose
3. Right Patient
4. Right Route
5. Right Time

When designing inpatient medication delivery systems, each of these aspects should be evaluated to ensure proper medication use.

A cornerstone of building a culture of safety for any hospital requires close attention to medication errors and systems design to prevent them. Simplifying and standardizing drugs and dosages to allow providers to be familiar with the formulary and the use of established drug protocols can avoid errors. Emphasis on medication reconciliation upon admission and discharge and improved patient education also will eliminate many of the common errors. There are many information technology applications for medication safety (88):

- Computerized Physician Order Entry—Studies have shown that CPOE streamlines the prescribing process and eliminates legibility issues. A high

percent of preventable ADEs are system related and can be mitigated with the use of sophisticated CPOE systems that have built-in clinical decision support, giving providers important, relevant information at the prescribing stage (87).

- Barcode/electronic medication administration technology (eMAR)—Barcode/eMAR systems match medication orders with drug products, provide verification of drugs at the dispensing and administration stages, and assist with automating the Five Rights of medication administration.
- Infusion pumps with "smart" technology—Intravenous medication administration systems with built-in smart technology assist clinicians by incorporating rules that apply to IV medication delivery (eg, dosing limits and clinical advisories) directly into the safety software of the infusion devices.
- Electronic prescribing—Electronic prescribing is described as writing a prescription with the use of a computer. Basic electronic prescribing systems ensure prescription completeness (avoiding errors of omission), whereas advanced electronic prescribing systems incorporate decision support tools into the prescribing process and can be electronically routed directly into pharmacy systems.
- Electronic health record—Use of an integrated comprehensive electronic health record that incorporates the patient's medication history and active medications is also an important technology aimed at preventing medication errors.

Medication ordering errors are the leading cause of preventable ADEs, and this aspect of medical care is within the control of each prescriber (89). These problems can be broken down into component elements with different systems corrections for each type of error.

- Medication order legibility—CPOE systems will virtually eliminate this problem.
- Missing medication order components—These errors can include the drug name, dosage, route of administration, and frequency. Again, CPOE systems can ensure the completeness of medication orders. Additionally, CPOE systems with built-in clinical decision supports can provide additional safety measures by providing alerts for drug allergies, drug–drug interactions, and dosing recommendations related to specific drug–patient characteristics such as age, weight, pregnancy, and renal function.
- Misuse of leading and trailing zeroes—The adage "always lead, never follow" can help mitigate errors, which can lead to 10-fold or 100-fold dosing errors.

- Inappropriate abbreviations—This topic is covered in a separate section of this chapter.
- *Pro re nata* (PRN or "as needed") medication orders—Common mistakes with these medications are often due to confusion with medications with similar names or are similar in appearance.
- Verbal medication orders—Most institutions limit use of verbal orders to urgent situations where written or electronic transmission is not possible. The importance of read-back orders is critical in these instances to prevent these mistakes.

Medication reconciliation systems are essential to the proper use of medications. One study showed a 42% incidence of medication continuity errors (defined as a discharge medication that is recorded in a patient's inpatient medical record but does not appear on the medication list at the first follow-up visit) for hospitalized patients (90). Researchers evaluated an inpatient computerized medication reconciliation tool. In this study, 65% of responders who used the system agreed that medication reconciliation improves patient care (91). A formal electronic medical record accessible to both inpatient and outpatient providers can eliminate these errors; however, even the simple use of a properly completed paper reconciliation form for each admission can also mitigate these errors. Noting the importance of this issue, the Joint Commission has established a National Patient Safety Goal 8 requiring hospitals to reconcile medications during transitions in care.

Use of sophisticated technology will help, but is not required, to reduce the current incidence of medication errors. According to the College's Committee on Quality Improvement and Patient Safety "focusing on elements that may prevent prescription errors and helping patients understand how to use prescribed medication properly may help lower the occurrence of medication use errors" (89).

Patient education is another essential element in eliminating medication errors. Patients and family members involved in their care must be given explicit and understandable directions about proper medication use. Understanding a patient's literacy is also critical when providing instructions. Patient understanding of why the medication is prescribed and the importance of taking it properly will lead to fewer patient errors. Having the patient maintain an up-to-date medication list that she can bring to all health care encounters is also helpful.

Hand Hygiene

It is estimated that approximately 90,000 hospital patient deaths per year are related to nosocomial infections. Many of these infections are considered preventable with proper attention to standard infection control guidelines and proper hand hygiene. An effective program of routine hand hygiene before and after every patient encounter for all caregivers is a critical component of a culture of safety. Effective infection control programs have been introduced in institutions around the country and have been proved to reduce the incidence of nosocomial infections and to be cost-effective. However, many institutions nationwide have been frustrated in their inability to establish a routine of hand hygiene for all physicians and nursing staff, despite evidence of the success of such programs.

The term hand hygiene includes either hand washing with soap and water or the use of alcohol-based gels or foams that do not require water. The introduction of alcohol-based products has made hand hygiene much easier to perform and less time consuming, leading to improved compliance with guidelines. The widespread placement of gel or foam dispensers in all patient care areas has made compliance much more successful and more likely to occur. Most infection control specialists recommend the use of alcohol-based hand rubs over soap and water hand washing at a sink because of improved compliance and more effective hand cleansing. However, the alcohol-based hand antiseptics are not effective for hands that are visibly dirty or those contaminated with organic materials (92).

Proper infection control programs, including hand hygiene guidelines, have become a requirement for Joint Commission hospital accreditation. The Joint Commission Standard IC.4.10 requires a routine of proper hand hygiene. In addition, the Joint Commission's National Patient Safety Goal 7 requires compliance with current World Health Organization (WHO) or Centers for Disease Control and Prevention (CDC) hand hygiene guidelines. Other organizations have endorsed effective hand washing guidelines, including the American Medical Association, the American Academy of Family Physicians (4 principles of hand awareness), the Agency for Healthcare Research and Quality, the Institute for Healthcare Improvement, and the College's *Guidelines for Perinatal Care*. The critical importance of proper hand hygiene, especially for prevention of methicillin-resistant *Staphylococcus aureus* (MRSA), is well-known and documented throughout the medical literature.

There are numerous suggestions that have been found to help improve hand hygiene campaigns in hospitals across the country. A hand awareness program may include posters, buttons, lapel pins, stickers, posted signs at every sink, and frequent reminders for all members of the health care team. Some institutions have encouraged patient involvement with information in every patient care area asking patients to remind caregivers to cleanse their hands before and after each patient contact, especially with systems of "gel in, gel out," utilizing convenient hand sanitizer dispensers in every patient care location.

The use of sterile or nonsterile gloves is also important in preventing serious hospital infections. Important reasons for the routine use of gloves for hospital personnel include the following:

- Providing an effective barrier between contaminated material or contaminated equipment and the caregiver's hands

- Reducing the likelihood of acquiring an infectious organism from a patient who is already colonized or infected with a known pathogen

- Preventing the transmission of a skin-carried pathogenic organism from hospital staff to patients

The use of gloves does not mean that proper hand hygiene can be omitted, as there can be defects or tears in gloves and skin can become contaminated when gloves are removed. Studies have demonstrated that organisms such as MRSA can still be recovered from a surgeon's hands after the gloves have been removed. Consequently, routine hand washing before and immediately after the use of gloves is required.

Overwhelming data supports the importance of proper hand hygiene; this must be a cornerstone of any hospital patient safety program. According to the *Guidelines for Perinatal Care, 6th edition*, "proper hand hygiene before and after each patient contact remains the single most important routine practice in the control of health care associated infections in both mother and neonate" (93).

Use of Abbreviations

Proper communication is essential for patient safety and important in preventing medical errors. One common source of errors is related to illegible handwriting; electronic medical records are helping to resolve this problem. Another important cause of adverse events, particularly medication errors, is the improper use of abbreviations.

In 2004, the Joint Commission published a list of "Do Not Use" abbreviations (Table 2-4), which has subsequently been reaffirmed (94). This list is now used by the Joint Commission for accreditation purposes during

Table 2-4. Joint Commission's Official "Do Not Use" List of Abbreviations[1]

Do Not Use	Potential Problem	Use Instead
U (unit)	Mistaken for "0" (zero), the number "4" (four) or "cc"	Write "unit"
IU (International Unit)	Mistaken for IV (intravenous) or the number 10 (ten)	Write "International Unit"
Q.D., QD, q.d., qd (daily)	Mistaken for each other	Write "daily"
Q.O.D., QOD, q.o.d, qod (every other day)	Period after the Q mistaken for "I" and the "O" mistaken for "I"	Write "every other day"
Trailing zero (X.0 mg)* Lack of leading zero (.X mg)	Decimal point is missed	Write X mg Write 0.X mg
MS	Can mean morphine sulfate or magnesium sulfate	Write "morphine sulfate"
MSO$_4$ and MgSO$_4$	Confused for one another	Write "magnesium sulfate"

[1]Applies to all orders and all medication-related documentation that is handwritten (including free-text computer entry) or on preprinted forms.

*Exception: A "trailing zero" may be used only where required to demonstrate the level of precision of the value being reported, such as for laboratory results, imaging studies that report size of lesions, or catheter and tube sizes. It may not be used in medication orders or other medication-related documentation.

Additional Abbreviations, Acronyms, and Symbols (For possible inclusion in the Official "Do Not Use" List)		
Do Not Use	**Potential Problem**	**Use Instead**
> (greater than) < (less than)	Misinterpreted as the number "7" (seven) or the letter "L" Confused for one another	Write "greater than" Write "less than"
Abbreviations for drug names	Misinterpreted due to similar abbreviations for multiple drugs	Write drug names in full
Apothecary units	Unfamiliar to many practitioners Confused with metric units	Use metric units
@	Mistaken for the number "2" (two)	Write "at"
cc	Mistaken for U (unit) when poorly written	Write "mL", "ml", or "milliliters" ("mL" is preferred)
μg	Mistaken for mg (milligrams) Results in one thousand-fold overdose	Write "mcg" or "micrograms"

© The Joint Commission 2009

their hospital reviews and has been one of the most frequent noncompliance findings in their surveys. The additional abbreviations listed are discouraged, but they are not currently used for accreditation purposes.

There are many abbreviations in common use at most institutions, but these can be confusing, have different meanings, or be improperly interpreted by other members of the health care team. The College's current recommendation states: "Because of the potential for ambiguity that might result in a medication error and subsequent patient harm, using fewer or perhaps no abbreviations is suggested" (95).

Disclosure of Adverse Events

Many health care professionals have found that disclosure of adverse events, if done properly, may actually defuse anger and possibly prevent litigation. Several national organizations, including the College, strongly encourage transparent communication with patients (96),

> Improving the disclosure process through policies, programmatic training, and accessible resources will enhance patient satisfaction, strengthen the physician–patient relationship, and most importantly, promote a higher quality of care.

Much can be learned by an institution from tracking both adverse events and near misses. An adverse event may be defined as a negative or unexpected result stemming from a diagnostic test, medical judgment or treatment, surgical intervention, or from the failure to perform a test, treatment, or intervention. It is not necessarily the result of medical error or professional negligence (97). A near miss is an error which could have caused harm, but did not, either by chance or timely intervention. It is the responsibility of the physician, perhaps in consultation with appropriate hospital administration, to decide if the severity of the event would warrant a formal disclosure session. Disclosing medical errors respects patient autonomy and is strongly desired by patients, and it has been endorsed by medical ethicists and numerous professional organizations.

Disclosure and Apology

It is important to recognize the distinction between disclosure and apology. More than one half of states have "apology laws" with very different terminoogy, protections, and specific statutes, and it is important for health care providers to know what is protected in their states. Disclosure is defined as providing information to a patient and/or family member about any incident while conveying a sense of openness and reciprocity. Apology acknowledges responsibility for an event coupled with an expression of remorse. Empathy and sympathy, an acknowledgement of suffering, are always appropriate and will strengthen the physician–patient bond.

Disclosure is no longer just an ethical imperative. It is a legal requirement in many states and is now mandated by the Joint Commission in Standard RI.290 (March 2007), which states, "patients, and when appropriate, their families, are informed about the outcomes of care, treatment and services that have been provided, including unanticipated outcomes." The standard represents a shift from mere endorsement of disclosure to a requirement for the hospital accreditation process. It also makes it clear that it is the responsibility of the primary practitioner (or designee) to inform the patient of the unanticipated outcome of care, but it does not describe the specific mechanics of how to proceed with the disclosure process. Many other national organizations also advocate for proper disclosure of adverse events, including the American Medical Association (Code of Medical Ethics Section 8.12), the National Patient Safety Foundation, and the College. According to the College (96),

> ... health care institutions should have written policies that address the timing, content, communication and documentation of disclosure. Once policies are developed, health care organizations should educate their providers on the policies and consider the need for additional resources and training.

Practitioners are strongly advised to consult with the hospital risk manager and their professional liability insurance carrier before proceeding with a formal disclosure. Many practitioners may not be familiar with the current state laws about disclosure, and it may be very helpful to be counseled before the disclosure occurs. If possible, establish the facts of the events and try to avoid speculating or offering opinions about causation of the event until all information is known. Most importantly, avoid blaming the patient or other health care providers involved in the patient's care. Always consider the health literacy and cultural issues of the specific patient and address patient privacy needs and concerns. Timeliness is important, and the discussion should be held as close to the event occurrence as is practical, usually within 48 hours.

There are many barriers to full disclosure, such as an overpowering sense of shame or guilt by the practitioner. Fear of litigation or disciplinary action also may prevent open communication with a patient. However, some studies suggest that patients expect and desire honest and open disclosure of an adverse event and are more likely to pursue litigation if they perceive that proper disclosure did not occur. Other studies have suggested that patients are spurred to legal action by a suspicion of a cover-up or a sense that full information has not been disclosed.

Many health care organizations have found that proper disclosure can lower litigation costs and reduce defensive medicine costs. The University of Michigan Health Systems has reported more than a 50% reduction in lawsuits and legal fees since implementing a policy of disclosure and apology in 2001. The Veteran Affairs Medical Center in Lexington, Kentucky, also has reported substantial litigation savings due to a program of full disclosure of medical errors. COPIC Insurance Company, the primary liability carrier in Colorado, has demonstrated significant legal savings from their 3Rs Program, to Recognize, Respond, and Resolve unanticipated medical events (98).

With the IOM report *To Err is Human: Building a Safer Health System*, medical errors gained increased attention. As a result, methods of managing and communicating about medical errors and unanticipated outcomes also gained increased focus. The disclosure of unanticipated outcomes with and without error is now mandatory in many states and is a common expectation. In fact, the Joint Commission Standard R1.2.90 requires that "patients, and when appropriate, their families are informed about the events of care, treatment, and services that have been provided." This standard also requires that "the responsible licensed independent practitioner or his or her designee informs the patient (and when appropriate, the family) about those unanticipated outcomes of care, treatment, and services" (99).

It is imperative that residency education recognize the existence of unanticipated outcomes and medical errors and incorporate disclosure and communication of these outcomes into training (ACGME competency of communication). Communication is a learned skill and disclosure conversations are an essential part of the resident training experience. This training will prepare residents for managing such conversations as attending physicians. Residents also should actively participate in regular M&M conferences, as this will assist them in central analysis of quality of care and potential areas for future improvement. In addition to observing disclosure conversations between attending physicians, hospital risk management and legal staff, and patients, residents need to receive formalized training on how to handle situations of medical errors and practice disclosure conversations. Residency training should address the concept of apologizing to a patient. Each residency program should adhere to respective state policy on the admissibility of disclosure and medical apology guidelines.

Currently, physicians often do not give full disclosure about medical errors, citing the following as barriers to disclosure: fear of litigation, fear of disciplinary actions, impact on future career, deficiency in communication skills, and working in the medical culture of infallibility. It is essential that residency education address these barriers and help residents develop both communication skills and skills in disclosure.

Disclosure and the Second Victim

Another effect of medical errors on health care providers is the concept of the "Second Victim," a term coined by Albert Wu, MD (100). The assumption is the first victim is the patient and patient's family. The second victim is the physician and health care provider team. It is crucial that residency programs recognize that all health care providers, especially trainees, can be negatively affected when involved in medical errors or even adverse outcomes that were not caused by medical error.

Ironically, enhanced communication, openness, and disclosure of medical errors are emphasized when referencing the patient and family. However, health care providers are encouraged, at times required, to not discuss the case. Involvement in medical errors can leave health care providers with guilt, shame, isolation, self-doubt, and fear of losing their job, reputation, and career. These emotions and perceptions can be magnified in residents. Resultant reactions can be burnout, depression, hyperdefensiveness, blame shifting, leaving medicine, mood changes, and suicide.

As humans, all people make mistakes. However, the expectation for physicians—real or perceived—is that there is no room for mistakes in the practice of modern medicine. Perfection is expected. This attitude does not facilitate education, during which trainees will make mistakes.

For residents and attending physicians, the mechanisms available to them following a medical error include presenting during morning reports, M&M conferences, and meetings of the quality improvement committee, and, when appropriate, conducting a root cause analysis. Every effort should be made to avoid the "Name-Blame-Shame game," avoiding the tendency to blame individuals for errors rather than looking at the root cause of an error. In fact, it might be helpful to consider that human errors are opportunities—not for shame or guilt—but for forgiveness, growth, and improvement in systems-based practices.

Because the impact of errors on health care providers can be significant, it is important to minimize the damage that they cause. The first step is to focus on prevention. Obviously, an error avoided is a recovery process that never needs to begin. If an error does occur, however, accepting responsibility is crucial. A logical follow-up might be pursuing additional training to better understand and correct mistakes. It is also important for physicians to understand that the need for support after an error is normal, not a sign of weakness. A common coping mechanism is discussion with colleagues and family members. Sources of support may also come from within a clinician's professional and social network, but may also include error disclosure to patients and family members.

The way that patients process medical errors includes the disclosure process itself, which should include an explanation of the error. Additional support available to patients includes their family and friends, resources at the hospital level, and legal support, if appropriate.

We should realize, however, that the existence of support for patients as first victims may never diminish the impact of medical error nor address the needs of the second victim.

A new approach for the processing of medical errors relates to a different paradigm for M&M review. The M&M review would be framed differently to include error acknowledgement (both system and individual), with particular attention to not just the clinical effect of an error, but also the personal effect.

Institutional support also is needed in processing medical errors. This would involve including material in education curriculum about reporting medical errors and disclosure, the use of employee assistance programs, one-on-one peer support, and the use of "confessor" figures, individuals with whom physicians can discuss errors confidentially. The program director, program chair, and all faculty must also support this new paradigm. The residency director who is responsible for resident evaluations may not be the best person to select as a confessor figure.

No one wants to have a medical error occur. However, when an error occurs, it is important to involve all participants in the process of examining the event, including the patient and her family. In examining the error, one must be proactive without creating a sense of isolation. It is also important to avoid the conspiracy of silence. For the health care provider, it is critical to survive the event intact, both professionally and personally.

Finally, it is incumbent on the program director, chair, faculty, and the Graduate Medical Education Committee to provide education on medical errors. It is also important to provide advice on error prevention and include residents in the review process of medical errors. Most importantly, the program director and others must provide emotional support and validate the feelings of any residents who have been involved in medical errors.

References

1. Hines S, Luna K, Lofthus J, Marquardt M, Stelmokas D. Becoming a high reliability organization: operational advice for hospital leaders. (Prepared by the Lewin Group under Contract No. 290-04-0011). AHRQ Publication No. 08-0022. Rockville (MD): AHRQ; 2008. Available at: http://www.ahrq.gov/QUAL/hroadvice/hroadvice.pdf. Retrieved June 9, 2009.

2. Kotter JP. Leading change. Boston (MA): Harvard Business School Press; 1996.

3. Parsons ML, Purdon TF, Craig B. Restructured quality and utilization management. In: Parsons ML, Murdaugh CL, Purdon TF, Jarrell BE, editors. Guide to clinical resource management. Gaithersburg (MD): Aspen Publishers; 1997. p. 16–33.

4. McEachern JE, Lord JT. The role of physicians in prioritizing the work of teams and the organization. In: Burton R, editor. The physician leader's guide. 2nd ed. Alexandria (VA): Capitol Publications; 1998. p. 27–40.

5. Center for Army Leadership. The U.S. Army leadership field manual: battle-tested wisdom for leaders in any organization. New York (NY): McGraw-Hill; 2004.

6. American College of Obstetricians and Gynecologists. Guidelines for Women's Health Care. 3 ed. Washington, DC: ACOG; 2007.

7. Lencioni P. The five dysfunctions of a team: a leadership fable. San Francisco (CA): Jossey-Bass; 2002.

8. Singer SJ, Tucker AL. Creating a culture of safety in hospitals. Briarcliff Manor (NY): Academy of Management; 2005. Available at: http://iis-db.stanford.edu/evnts/4218/Creating_Safety_Culture-SSingerRIP.pdf. Retrieved June 9, 2009.

9. Accreditation Council for Graduate Medical Education. Common program requirements: general competencies. Chicago (IL): ACGME; 2007. Available at: http://www.acgme.org/outcome/comp/GeneralCompetenciesStandards21307.pdf. Retrieved June 9, 2009.

10. The Joint Commission. 2009 national patient safety goals. Oakbrook Terrace (IL): JC; 2009. Available at: http://www.jointcommission.org/PatientSafety/NationalPatientSafetyGoals. Retrieved June 2, 2009.

11. The Joint Commission. Comprehensive accreditation manual. CAMH for hospitals: the official handbook. Oakbrook Terrace (IL): JC; 2009.

12. Juran D. Achieving sustained quantifiable results in an interdepartmental quality improvement project. Jt Comm J Qual Improv 1994;20:105–19.

13. Berwick DM, Godfrey AB, Roessner J. Using the scientific method to define problems. In: Curing healthcare: new strategies for quality improvement: a report on the National Demonstration Project on Quality Improvement in Health Care. San Francisco (CA): Jossey-Bass; 1990. p. 46–66.

14. Take the lead out of quality improvement projects. Hosp Peer Rev 1996;21:19,20,33,34.

15. Berwick DM, Godfrey AB, Roessner J. Resource C: three project reports. In: Curing health care: new strategies for quality improvement: a report on the National Demonstration Project on Quality Improvement in Health Care. San Francisco (CA): Jossey-Bass; 1990. p. 221–74.

16. Institute for Healthcare Improvement. A step-by-step guide to reducing cesarean section rates. In: Reducing cesarean section rates while maintaining maternal and infant outcomes. Boston (MA): IHI; 1997. p. 13–35.

17. Brennan TA. Physician's professional responsibility to improve the quality of care. Acad Med 2002;77:973–80.

18. Bradley EH, Holmboe ES, Mattera JA, Roumanis SA, Radford MJ, Krumholz HM. A qualitative study of increasing beta-blocker use after myocardial infarction: why do some hospitals succeed? JAMA 2001;285:2604–11.

19. Nelson EC, Splaine ME, Plume SK, Batalden P. Good measurement for good improvement work. Qual Manag Health Care 2004;13:1–16.

20. Hamby LS, Colacchio TA, Nelson EC. Application of quality improvement to surgical practice. Surgery 2000;128:836–44.

21. Nelson EC, Splaine ME, Batalden PB, Plume SK. Building measurement and data collection into medical practice. Ann Intern Med 1998;128:460–6.

22. Jones ML, Day S, Creely J, Woodland MB, Gerdes JB. Implementation of a clinical pathway system in maternal newborn care: a comprehensive documentation system for outcomes management. J Perinat Neonatal Nurs 1999;13:1–20.

23. Darby M. 12 ways to get physician buy-in to practice guidelines. Qual Lett Healthc Lead 1998;10:2–8.

24. Marshall M, Campbell S, Hacker J, Roland M, editors. Quality indicators for general practice: a practical guide for health professionals and managers. London (UK): Royal Society of Medicine Press; 2002.

25. Mainz J. Defining and classifying clinical indicators for quality improvement. Int J Qual Health Care 2003;15:523–30.

26. Donabedian A. Evaluating the quality of medical care. Milbank Mem Fund Q 1966;44(suppl):166–206.

27. Palmer RH, Reilly MC. Individual and institutional variables which may serve as indicators of quality of medical care. Med Care 1979;17:693–717.

28. Palmer RH. Using health outcomes data to compare plans, networks and providers. Int J Qual Health Care 1998;10:477–83.

29. Agency for Healthcare Research and Quality. Guide to prevention quality indicators: hospital admission for ambulatory care sensitive conditions. Version 3.1. Rockville (MD): AHRQ; 2007. Available at: http://www.qualityindicators.ahrq.gov/downloads/pqi/pqi_guide_v31.pdf. Retrieved June 9, 2009.

30. Mainz J. Developing evidence-based clinical indicators: a state of the art methods primer. Int J Qual Health Care 2003;15(suppl 1):i5–11.

31. Institute of Medicine (US). Crossing the quality chasm: a new health system for the 21st century. Washington, DC: National Academy Press; 2001.

32. Mann S, Pratt S, Gluck P, Nielsen P, Risser D, Greenberg P, et al. Assessing quality obstetrical care: development of standardized measures. Jt Comm J Qual Patient Saf 2006;32:497–505.

33. Nielsen PE, Goldman MB, Mann S, Shapiro DE, Marcus RG, Pratt SD, et al. Effects of teamwork training on adverse outcomes and process of care in labor and delivery: a randomized controlled trial. Obstet Gynecol 2007;109:48–55.

34. Institute of Medicine (US). Performance measurement: accelerating improvement. Washington, DC: National Academies Press; 2006.

35. Lilford RJ, Brown CA, Nicholl J. Use of process measures to monitor the quality of clinical practice. BMJ 2007;335:648–50.

36. National Practitioner Data Bank, Healthcare Integrity and Protection Data Bank. Fact sheet on the National Practitioner Data Bank. Rockville (MD): NPDB-HIPDB; 2008. Available at: http://npdb-hipdb.com/pubs/fs/Fact_Sheet-National_Practitioner_Data_Bank.pdf. Retrieved June 9, 2009.

37. Hospitals now required to evaluate physicians continuously. ACOG Today 2008;52(1):7.

38. Briggs LA, Heath J, Kelley J. Peer review for advanced practice nurses: what does it really mean? AACN Clin Issues 2005;16:3–15.

39. Sheahan SL, Simpson C, Rayens MK. Nurse practitioner peer review: process and evaluation. J Am Acad Nurse Pract 2001;13:140–5.

40. Goldman RL. The reliability of peer assessments of quality of care. JAMA 1992;267:958–60.

41. Violato C, Marini A, Toews J, Lockyer J, Fidler H. Feasibility and psychometric properties of using peers, consulting physicians, co-workers, and patients to assess physicians. Acad Med 1997;72:S82–4.

42. Ramsey PG, Wenrich MD, Carline JD, Inui TS, Larson EB, LoGerfo JP. Use of peer ratings to evaluate physician performance. JAMA 1993;269:1655–60.

43. Ramsey PG, Wenrich MD. Peer ratings. An assessment tool whose time has come. J Gen Intern Med 1999;14:581-2.

44. McLeod PJ, Tamblyn R, Benaroya S, Snell L. Faculty ratings of resident humanism predict patient satisfaction ratings in ambulatory medical clinics. J Gen Intern Med 1994;9:321–6.

45. Woolliscroft JO, Howell JD, Patel BP, Swanson DB. Resident-patient interactions: the humanistic qualities of internal medicine residents assessed by patients, attending physicians, program supervisors, and nurses. Acad Med 1994;69:216–24.

46. Goldman RL. The reliability of peer assessments. A meta-analysis. Eval Health Prof 1994;17:3–21.

47. Evans R, Elwyn G, Edwards A. Review of instruments for peer assessment of physicians. BMJ 2004;328:1240.

48. Ramsey PG, Carline JD, Blank LL, Wenrich MD. Feasibility of hospital-based use of peer ratings to evaluate the performances of practicing physicians. Acad Med 1996;71:364–70.

49. Lipner RS, Blank LL, Leas BF, Fortna GS. The value of patient and peer ratings in recertification. Acad Med 2002;77(suppl):S64–6.

50. Hall W, Violato C, Lewkonia R, Lockyer J, Fidler H, Toews J, et al. Assessment of physician performance in Alberta: the physician achievement review. CMAJ 1999;161:52–7.

51. Thomas PA, Gebo KA, Hellmann DB. A pilot study of peer review in residency training. J Gen Intern Med 1999;14:551–4.

52. Disruptive behavior. ACOG Committee Opinion No. 366. American College of Obstetricians and Gynecologists. Obstet Gynecol 2007;109:1261–2.

53. Steiger B. Special report: quality of care survey. Doctors say many obstacles block paths to patient safety. Physician Exec 2007;33(3):6–14.

54. Frankel A, Graydon-Baker E, Neppl C, Simmonds T, Gustafson M, Gandhi TK. Patient safety leadership WalkRounds. Jt Comm J Qual Saf 2003;29:16–26.

55. Kotter J, Rathgeber H. Our iceberg is melting: changing and succeeding under any conditions. New York (NY): St. Martin's Press; 2006.

56. Laffel G, Blumenthal D. The case for using industrial quality management science in health care organizations. JAMA 1989;262:2869–73.

57. Lichtmacher A. Quality assessment tools: ACOG Voluntary Review of Quality of Care Program, Peer Review Reporting System. Obstet Gynecol Clin North Am 2008;35:147–62, x.

58. Cherouny PH, Federico FA, Haraden C, Leavitt Gullo S, Resar R. Idealized design of perinatal care. IHI Innovation Series white paper. Cambridge (MA): Institute for Healthcare Improvement; 2005.

59. Salus Global Corporation. The MORE^OB program: Managing Obstetrical Risk Efficiently. Available at: http://www.salusgc.com/moreob_overview.html. Retrieved June 9, 2009.

60. Press Ganey Associates. Safety culture: staff perspectives on American health care. Pulse Report 2009. South Bend (IN): Press Ganey; 2009. Available at: http://www.pressganey.com/galleries/default-file/Safety_Culture_Pulse_Report_2009.pdf. Retrieved June 9, 2009.

61. Centers for Medicare and Medicaid Services. Hospital Consumer Assessment of Healthcare Providers and Systems: CAHPS® hospital survey. Baltimore (MD): CMS; 2009. Available at: http://www.hcahpsonline.org/home.aspx. Retrieved June 9, 2009.

62. U.S. Department of Health and Human Services. Hospital compare: a quality tool provided by Medicare. Washington, DC: DHHS; 2009. Available at: http://www.hospitalcompare.hhs.gov. Retrieved June 10, 2009.

63. Agency for Healthcare Research and Quality. Conclusions and recommendations. In: Medical teamwork and patient safety: the evidence-based relation. AHRQ Publication No. 05-0053. Rockville (MD): AHRQ; 2005. p. 43–8. Available at http://www.ahrq.gov/qual/medteam/medteam5.pdf. Retrieved June 10, 2009.

64. Nova. The deadliest plane crash: the final eight minutes. Boston (MA): WGBH Educational Foundation; 2006. Available at: http://www.pbs.org/wgbh/nova/planecrash/minutes.html. Retrieved June 10, 2009.

65. Helmreich RL, Merritt AC, Wilhelm JA. The evolution of Crew Resource Management training in commercial aviation. Int J Aviat Psychol 1999;9:19–32.

66. Joint Commission on Accreditation of Healthcare Organizations. Health care at the crossroads: strategies for improving the medical liability system and preventing patient injury. Oakbrook Terrace (IL): JC; 2005. Available at: http://www.jointcommission.org/NR/rdonlyres/167DD821-A395-48FD-87F9-6AB12BCACB0F/0/Medical_Liability.pdf. Retrieved June 12, 2009.

67. The Joint Commission. Preventing infant death and injury during delivery. Sentinel Event Alert Issue No. 30. Oakbrook Terrace (IL): JC; 2004. Available at: http://www.jointcommission.org/SentinelEvents/SentinelEventAlert/sea_30.htm. Retrieved June 12, 2009.

68. Naik G. New formula: A hospital races to learn lessons of Ferrari pit stop. Wall Street Journal. November 14, 2006:A1.

69. Hashimoto H, Bohmer RM, Harrell LC, Palacios IF. Continuous quality improvement decreases length of stay and adverse events: a case study in an interventional cardiology program. Am J Manag Care 1997;3:1141–50.

70. Bodenheimer T. Building teams in primary care: lessons from 15 case studies. Oakland (CA): California HealthCare Foundation; 2007. Available at: http://www.chcf.org/topics/chronicdisease/index.cfm?itemID=133375. Retrieved June 12, 2009.

71. Wise H, Beckhard R, Rubin I, Kyte A. Making health teams work. Cambridge (MA): Ballinger; 1974.

72. Mann S, Marcus R, Sachs B. Lessons from the cockpit: how team training can reduce errors on L&D. Contemp OB/GYN 2006;51(1):34–45.

73. Agency for Healthcare Research and Quality. Team STEPPS™: national implementation. Available at: http://teamstepps.ahrq.gov/index.htm. Retrieved June 12, 2009.

74. The Joint Commission. Sentinel event root cause and trend data. In: Improving America's hospitals: the Joint Commission's annual report on quality and safety 2007. Oakbrook Terrace (IL): JC; 2007. p. 45–8. Available at: http://www.jointcommissionreport.org/pdf/JC_2007_Annual_report.pdf. Retrieved June 12, 2009.

75. Leonard M, Graham S, Bonacum D. The human factor: the critical importance of effective teamwork and communication in providing safe care. Qual Saf Health Care 2004;13(suppl 1):i85–i90.

76. Agency for Healthcare Research and Quality. Patient safety culture surveys. Rockville (MD): AHRQ; 2009. Available at: http://www.ahrq.gov/qual/patientsafetyculture. Retrieved June 12, 2009.

77. Agency for Healthcare Research and Quality. Is your organization ready for TeamSTEPPS? Available at: http://teamstepps.ahrq.gov/ahrqchecklist.aspx. Retrieved June 12, 2009.

78. Nielsen PE, Goldman MB, Mann S, Shapiro DE, Marcus RG, Pratt SD, et al. Effects of teamwork training on adverse outcomes and process of care in labor and delivery: a randomized controlled trial. Obstet Gynecol 2007;109:48–55.

79. Bodenheimer T, Grumbach K. Improving primary care: strategies and tools for a better practice. New York (NY): Lange Medical Books/McGraw-Hill; 2007.

80. Risser DT, Rice MM, Salisbury ML, Simon R, Jay GD, Berns SD. The potential for improved teamwork to reduce medical errors in the emergency department. The MedTeams Research Consortium. Ann Emerg Med 1999;34:373–83.

81. Laurant MG, Hermens RP, Braspenning JC, Sibbald B, Grol RP. Impact of nurse practitioners on workload of general practitioners: randomised controlled trial. BMJ 2004;328:927.

82. Patient safety in the surgical environment. ACOG Committee Opinion No. 328. American College of Obstetricians and Gynecologists. Obstet Gynecol 2006;107:429–33.

83. The Joint Commission. Universal protocol for preventing wrong site, wrong procedure, wrong person surgery. Oakbrook Terrace (IL): JC; 2009. Available at: http://www.jointcommission.org/PatientSafety/UniversalProtocol. Retrieved June 10, 2009.

84. Accreditation Council for Graduate Medical Education. Common program requirements: general competencies. Chicago (IL): ACGME; 2007. Available at: http://www.acgme.org/outcome/comp/GeneralCompetenciesStandards 21307.pdf. Retrieved June 9, 2009.

85. Charles C, Gafni A, Whelan T. Shared decision-making in the medical encounter: what does it mean? (or it takes at least two to tango). Soc Sci Med 1997;44:681–92.

86. Bates DW, Cullen DJ, Laird N, Petersen LA, Small SD, Servi D, et al. Incidence of adverse drug events and potential adverse drug events. Implications for prevention. ADE Prevention Study Group. JAMA 1995;274:29–34.

87. Institute of Medicine (US). Preventing medication errors. Washington, DC: National Academies Press; 2007.

88. Technologic advances to reduce medication-related errors. ACOG Committee Opinion No. 400. American College of Obstetricians and Gynecologists. Obstet Gynecol 2008;111:795–8.

89. Safe use of medication. ACOG Committee Opinion No. 331. American College of Obstetricians and Gynecologists. Obstet Gynecol 2006;107:969–72.

90. Moore C, Wisnivesky J, Williams S, McGinn T. Medical errors related to discontinuity of care from an inpatient to an outpatient setting. J Gen Intern Med 2003;18:646–51.

91. Turchin A, Hamann C, Schnipper JL, Graydon-Baker E, Millar SG, McCarthy PC, et al. Evaluation of an inpatient computerized medication reconciliation system. J Am Med Inform Assoc 2008;15:449–52.

92. Boyce JM, Pittet D. Guideline for hand hygiene in health-care settings. Recommendations of the Healthcare Infection Control Practices Advisory Committee and the HICPAC/SHEA/APIC/IDSA Hand Hygiene Task Force. Society for Healthcare Epidemiology of America/Association for Professionals in Infection Control/Infectious Diseases Society of America. MMWR Recomm Rep 2002;51:1–45, quiz CE1-4. Available at: http://www.cdc.gov/mmwr/PDF/rr/rr5116.pdf. Retrieved June 10, 2009.

93. American Academy of Pediatrics, American College of Obstetricians and Gynecologists. Guidelines for perinatal

care. 6th ed. Elk Grove Village (IL): AAP; Washington, DC: ACOG; 2007.

94. The Joint Commission. The official "do not use" list. Oakbrook Terrace (IL): JC; 2009. Available at: http://www. jointcommission.org/NR/rdonlyres/2329F8F5-6EC5-4E21-B932-54B2B7D53F00/0/dnu_list.pdf. Retrieved June 10, 2009.

95. "Do not use" abbreviations. ACOG Committee Opinion No. 327. American College of Obstetricians and Gynecologists. Obstet Gynecol 2006;107:213–4.

96. Disclosure and discussion of adverse events. ACOG Committee Opinion No. 380. American College of Obstetricians and Gynecologists. Obstet Gynecol 2007;110:957–8.

97. Managing the risks of an unanticipated outcome, before, during and after the event. Norcal Mutual Insurance Company. Claims RX. May 2007:1–11.

98. COPIC Companies. 3Rs program. Denver (CO): COPIC Companies; 2009. Available at: http://www.callcopic.com/home/what-we-offer/coverages/medical-professional-liability-insurance-ne/physicians-medical-practices/special-programs/3rs-program/. Retrieved June 10, 2009.

99. The Joint Commission. Comprehensive accreditation manual. CAMH for hospitals: the official handbook. Oakbrook Terrace (IL): JC; 2009.

100. Wu AW. Medical error: the second victim. The doctor who makes the mistake needs help too. BMJ 2000;320:726–7.

PART 3

Assessing Clinical Competence

Credentialing and granting privileges to members of its medical staff are among the most important responsibilities of any health care facility. Credentialing is a multifaceted process that involves verification of licensure, education and training, malpractice experience, malpractice insurance coverage, and board certification as required by the facility. It requires that reports are requested from the National Practitioner Data Bank and other facilities where the applicant has or has had privileges.

The more difficult, yet critical, aspect of this process is determining which requested privileges will be granted. Privileging defines what procedures a credentialed practitioner is permitted to perform at the facility. The granting of privileges is based on training, experience, and demonstrated current clinical competence. Each staff member must be assessed at the time of initial application as well as every 2 years at the time of reappraisal. In addition to routine requests for privileges, a physician also may request privileges to perform a new technology. The process of assessing current clinical competence and granting privileges is difficult and time-consuming, yet it is a critically necessary activity.

Although the terms "credentialing" and "privileging" often are used interchangeably, they are different processes. Credentialing assures membership and comprises the aforementioned components. For privileging, there have been various approaches to setting criteria, such as the following methods (1):

1. Laundry list method—An applicant can specifically request procedures and conditions from a checklist.
2. Categorization—Major procedures or treatment areas are identified and classified based on complexity or the level of training.
3. Descriptive—Allows the applicant to describe the requested privileges in narrative form.
4. Delineation by codes—Privileges are requested based on diagnosis codes from the *International Classification of Diseases, Ninth Revision, Clinical Modification*, procedure codes from *Current Procedural Terminology*, or grouping codes from Diagnosis-Related Group codes.
5. Combination—A hybrid of two or more of the methods described.
6. Core privileging—An alternative to the methods described. This assumes that anyone who has completed an approved residency has sufficient knowledge and technical skills to perform competently within the specialty. This method allows for consistency, flexibility, and objective screening for all applicants.

Privileges often are formatted by levels (eg, Levels I, II, and III obstetric privileges and Levels I, II, and III gynecologic privileges). As new technologies evolve, processes for granting privileges for them will need to be formulated. For a sample application for privileges, which outlines such areas as emergency situations, provisional period, and the performance of new procedures, see Appendix F. Hospitals using these materials may adapt them to conform to the specific situations at these facilities. This information is not intended to be all inclusive or exclusive. It is intended primarily for educational purposes.

Granting Privileges

The following list has been developed to aid in granting privileges to those health care providers within the facility to perform obstetric and gynecologic procedures. The granting of privileges at any level in obstetrics and gynecology is based on satisfaction of criteria for the specified procedures. Criteria for granting privileges must be applied consistently regardless of the applicant's specialty. As stated, the granting of clinical privileges must be based on training, experience, and demonstrated current clinical competence. The educational requirements assume that applicants have achieved a doctor of medicine or doctor of osteopathy degree. Except as otherwise noted, prerequisites for each category of privileges are listed as follows:

Training

- Successful completion of an Accreditation Council for Continuing Medical Education (ACGME)-accredited residency program in obstetrics–gynecology

Certification

- Board certification (or active candidate) by the American Board of Obstetrics and Gynecology or the American Osteopathic Board of Obstetrics and Gynecology
- Maintenance of Certification, if applicable

Reappraisal (recredentialing/reprivileging) (2-year cycle) should require:

- Review of quality improvement file:
  — trending
  — sentinel events
  — other problems with specific procedures
- Review of level of activity:
  — total number of cases
  — total number of complications
  — outcomes

- If the credentials committee determines that the number of cases performed within the cycle is insufficient for adequately assessing competency, it may recommend that the individual be proctored and evaluated for a designated period until competency is demonstrated. However, if the physician has privileges at another institution for the particular procedure, then the individual must provide credentialing data from that hospital for review by the credentials committee and may not require proctoring.

I. Obstetric Privileges

A. Level I (Basic) Obstetric Privileges
   1. Privileges may include:
      a. Management of labor
      b. Pudendal and local anesthesia
      c. Fetal assessment, antepartum and intrapartum, including limited obstetric ultrasound examination
      d. Induction of labor
      e. Internal fetal monitoring
      f. Normal cephalic delivery, including use of vacuum extraction and outlet forceps
      g. Episiotomy and repair, including third-degree lacerations
      h. Management of common intrapartum problems
      i. Exploration of vagina, cervix, and uterus
      j. Emergency breech delivery
      k. Management of common postpartum problems
      l. First-assist at cesarean delivery
      m. Circumcision

B. Level II (Specialty) Obstetric Privileges
   1. Privileges may include:
      a. All Level I obstetric privileges
      b. Management of normal and abnormal labor and delivery (including premature labor, breech presentation, cesarean delivery, vaginal delivery after previous cesarean delivery, cephalopelvic disproportion, non-reassuring fetal status, use of amniotomy and oxytocin, and midforceps delivery)
      c. Management of medical or surgical complications of pregnancy
      d. Diagnostic amniocentesis
      e. Cesarean hysterectomy
      f. Hypogastric artery ligation
      g. Vaginal cerclage or treatment of incompetent cervix
      h. External version of breech presentation
      i. Obstetric ultrasonography—complete
      j. Midforceps rotation
      k. Regional anesthesia as determined by training and local practice
   2. Board certification (or active candidate) by the American Board of Obstetrics and Gynecology in maternal–fetal medicine may be considered

C. Level III (Subspecialty) Obstetric Privileges
   1. Privileges may include:
      a. All Level I and II obstetric privileges
      b. Intrauterine fetal transfusion
      c. Intrauterine fetal surgery
      d. Chorionic villous sampling
      e. Percutaneous umbilical sampling
   2. Training should include documentation of specialized postresidency training
   3. Subspecialty certification (or active candidate) by the American Board of Obstetrics and Gynecology in maternal–fetal medicine may be considered

II. Gynecologic Privileges

A. Level I (Basic) Gynecologic Privileges

1. Privileges may include:

   a. Appropriate screening examination of the female, including breast examination

   b. Obtaining vaginal and cervical cytology

   c. Colposcopy

   d. Cervical biopsy, polypectomy

   e. Endometrial biopsy

   f. Cryosurgery/cautery for benign disease

   g. Microscopic diagnosis of urine and vaginal smears

   h. Bartholin cyst drainage or marsupialization

   i. Dilation and curettage for incomplete abortion

   j. Vulvar biopsy

B. Level II (Specialty) Gynecologic Privileges

1. Privileges may include:

   a. All Level I gynecologic privileges

   b. Dilation and curettage

   c. Dilation and curettage, with or without conization

   d. Laparotomy

   e. Operations for removal of uterus, cervix, oviducts, ovaries (abdominal or vaginal), and appendix

   f. Diagnostic laparoscopy

   g. Diagnostic hysteroscopy

   h. Tubal sterilization

   i. Operations for treatment of urinary stress incontinence, vaginal approach, retropubic urethral suspension, or sling procedure

   j. Fistula repairs (vesicovaginal or rectovaginal)

   k. Tuboplasty

   l. Hernia repair (incisional or umbilical)

   m. Operations for treatment of noninvasive carcinoma of vulva, vagina, uterus, ovary, and cervix

   n. Repair of rectocele, enterocele, cystocele

   o. Vaginectomy (total or partial)

   p. Colpocleisis

   q. Strassman procedure (metroplasty)

   r. Myomectomy

   s. Node dissection (superficial inguinal, pelvic, or paraaortic)

   t. Diagnostic hysteroscopy

   u. Second-trimester abortion by medical or surgical means

C. Level III-A: Basic Endoscopic Procedures

1. Privileges may include:

   a. All Level I and II gynecologic privileges

   b. Endoscopic ovarian or endometrial biopsy

   c. Minor adhesiolysis

   d. Management of ectopic pregnancy (linear salpingostomy, partial salpingectomy)

   e. Destruction of endometriosis stage I and stage II as graded by American Society of Reproductive Medicine criteria

2. Training should include successful completion of an ACGME-accredited residency program in obstetrics and gynecology

3. Certification should be required:

   a. Board certification (or active candidate) by the American Board of Obstetrics and Gynecology

   b. Maintenance of Certification, if applicable

4. Experience should be required:

   a. The applicant must possess the proficiency and be privileged to perform the requested procedures in an open (laparotomy) manner

   b. The applicant should have been granted privileges to perform basic (Level III-A) endoscopic procedures and should have demonstrated competency in these techniques

D. Level III-B: Advanced Endoscopic Procedures

1. Privileges may include:

   a. All Level I and II gynecologic privileges

   b. Laparoscopically assisted vaginal hysterectomy

   c. Ovarian cystectomy

   d. Salpingo-oophorectomy

   e. Adhesiolysis

   f. Management of endometriosis, stage III and IV

   g. Division of the uterosacral ligaments

   h. Appendectomy

   i. Operative hysteroscopy requiring use of the resectoscope (division or resection of the uterine septum, surgical treatment of Asherman's syndrome, resection of uterine myomas)

   j. Myomectomy

   k. Pelvic lymphadenectomy

   l. Pelvic sidewall dissection

   m. Ureteral dissection

n. Presacral neurectomy

o. Dissection of obliterated pouch of Douglas

p. Hernia repair

q. Retropubic bladder neck suspension

r. Sling procedure

s. Bowel surgery

t. Total hysterectomy

u. Supracervical hysterectomy

2. Also required is successful completion of advanced training that includes training in listed procedures, or documented course, including didactic and hands-on laboratory experience, unless included in residency program

3. Experience should include advanced procedures requiring the following additional training and documentation:

a. Completion of a postgraduate course, accredited by the ACCME that includes didactic training (must include education on equipment operation and safety factors) and hands-on laboratory experience, *and*

b. If the privileges requested were not included in residency training, the applicant must follow the requirements for a preceptorship as discussed under the section for "Requests for New Privileges."

c. In the event that credentials in advanced endoscopy are already established at a different hospital, the applicant must present evidence of these established credentials in lieu of (a) and (b) above. In addition, the applicant must provide a list of cases performed over the past 24 months, including preoperative and postoperative diagnoses, procedure, type of endoscope used, outcome, and complications of the procedure.

d. A letter from the director of an approved residency program can substitute for (a) and (b) above. In addition, this new residency graduate must provide a list of advanced endoscopy cases performed over the past 24 months.

E. Level III-C: Gynecologic Oncology

1. Privileges may include:

a. All Level I and II gynecologic privileges

b. Treatment of malignant disease with chemotherapy

c. Radical hysterectomy for treatment of invasive carcinoma of the cervix and uterus

d. Radical surgery for treatment of gynecologic malignancy to include procedures on bowel, ureter, bladder, pelvic or abdominal organs, as indicated

e. Treatment of invasive carcinoma of vulva by radical vulvectomy

f. Treatment of invasive carcinoma of the vagina by radical vaginectomy and other appropriate surgery

g. Pelvic, periaortic, and inguinal lymphadenectomy and reconstructive surgery of pelvis and external genitalia

2. Training should also include documentation of specialized postresidency training, experience, or subspecialty certification by the American Board of Obstetrics and Gynecology.

F. Level III-D: Assisted Reproductive Techniques

1. Privileges may include:

a. Gynecologic Levels I, II, III-A, and III-B

b. In vitro fertilization and gamete intrafallopian transfer

c. Monitoring of ovulation induction and intrauterine insemination

d. Management of ovarian hyperstimulation

2. Training should also include:

a. Documentation of training and experience in reproductive endocrinology and pelvic reproductive surgery, including experience in operative laparoscopic procedures, *and*

b. Documentation of training and experience with in vitro fertilization–embryo transfer and gamete intrafallopian transfer procedures.

3. Subspecialty certification (or active candidate) by the American Board of Obstetrics and Gynecology in reproductive endocrinology and infertility may also be considered.

4. Experience should require demonstrating knowledge of all aspects of assisted reproductive techniques.

G. Level III-E: Laser Therapy

1. Privileges may include:

a. Laser therapy for cervix, vagina, vulva, and perineum (colposcopically directed)

b. Conization of cervix

c. Lysis of adhesions and photocoagulation (intraabdominal "free hand use")

d. Lysis of adhesions and photocoagulation (microscopically directed)

e. Oncologic debulking procedures (intraabdominal "free hand use")

2. Training should also include:

a. Documentation of laser training from a residency program director, attesting to the completion of at least 8 hours of observation and hands-on involvement, *or*

b. Documentation of a laser training course, including laser physics, safety, indications and complications, and hands-on experience.

3. Experience should include:

a. Level II gynecologic privileges, *and*

b. Laser privileges as defined on the hospital-wide laser privilege request form

H. Level III-F: Endometrial Ablation

1. Privileges may include:

a. Laser ablation

b. Electrosurgical ablation

c. Thermal balloon ablation

d. Other techniques

2. Training should also include additional training for the following procedures:

a. Laser ablation

(1) Documentation from residency program director, attesting to hands-on involvement and competence, *or*

(2) Documentation of an operative hysteroscopy and laser ablation of the endometrium course, including laser physics, safety, indications and complications, and hands-on experience

b. Electrosurgical ablation

(1) Documentation from residency program director, including at least 8 hours of observation and hands-on involvement, *or*

(2) Documentation of competency and demonstration of hands-on experience in operative hysteroscopy with endometrial rollerball

c. Thermal balloon ablation

(1) Documentation from residency program director, attesting to the completion of at least 8 hours of observation and hands-on involvement, *or*

(2) Documentation of competency and demonstration of hands-on experience

3. Experience should include proficiency in diagnostic hysteroscopy if laser or electrosurgical ablation is performed

III. Credentialing for Family Physicians

A. Obstetric Privileges for Family Physicians

1. Privileges may include:

a. Management of labor

b. Pudendal and local block anesthesia

c. Fetal assessment, antepartum and intrapartum, including limited obstetric ultrasound examination

d. Internal fetal monitoring

e. Normal cephalic delivery

f. Management of common intrapartum problems

g. Exploration of vagina, cervix, and uterus

h. Emergency breech delivery

i. Management of common postpartum problems

j. First-assist at cesarean delivery

2. Family physicians requesting these privileges must demonstrate:

a. Successful completion of obstetric training as delineated in the special requirements for residency training in Family Medicine by the ACGME

b. If transferring from another institution, documentation of current competence as supported by ongoing clinical practice and quality review data

c. Maintenance of board certification (or active candidate) by the American Board of Family Physicians

B. Advanced Obstetric Privileges for Family Physicians

1. Privileges may include:

a. Operative vaginal delivery, including low forceps or vacuum extraction

b. Induction of labor

c. Management of high-risk pregnancy

2. Family physicians requesting these privileges must demonstrate:

a. Additional intensive experience taught by or in collaboration with obstetrician–gynecologists (2). In programs where obstetrician–gynecologists are not available, these skills should be taught by appropriately skilled and credentialed family physicians.

b. The assignment of hospital privileges is a local responsibility, and privileges should be granted on the basis of training, experience, and demonstrated current clinical competence. All physicians should be held to the same standards for granting privileges, regardless of specialty, in order to assure the provision of high-quality patient care. Prearranged, collaborative relationships should be established to ensure ongoing consultations, as well as consultations needed for emergencies.

The standard of training should allow any physician who receives training in a cognitive or surgical skill to meet the criteria for privileges in that area of practice. Provisional privileges in primary care, obstetric care, and cesarean delivery should be granted regardless of specialty as long as training criteria and experience are documented. All physicians should be subject to a proctorship period to allow demonstration of ability and current competence. These principles should apply to all health care systems.

   c. Privileges recommended by the department of family practice shall be the responsibility of the department of family practice. Similarly, privileges recommended by the department of obstetrics and gynecology shall be the responsibility of the department of obstetrics and gynecology. When privileges are recommended jointly by the departments of family practice and obstetrics and gynecology, they shall be the joint responsibility of the two departments.

C. Gynecologic Privileges for Family Physicians

   1. Privileges may include:

      a. Appropriate screening examination of the female, including breast examination

      b. Obtaining vaginal and cervical cytology

      c. Colposcopy

      d. Cervical biopsy, polypectomy

      e. Endometrial biopsy

      f. Cryosurgery/cautery for benign disease

      g. Microscopic diagnosis of urine and vaginal smears

      h. Bartholin duct cyst drainage or marsupialization

      i. Vulvar biopsy

   2. Family physicians requesting these privileges must demonstrate:

      a. Successful completion of gynecologic training as delineated in the special requirements for residency training in Family Medicine by the ACGME

      b. If transferring from another institution, documentation of current competence as supported by ongoing clinical practice and quality review data

      c. Maintenance of board certification (or active candidate) by the American Board of Family Medicine

Requests for New Privileges

New Equipment and Technology

New equipment or technology usually improves health care, provided that practitioners and other hospital staff understand the proper indications for usage. Problems can arise when staff perform duties or use equipment for which they are not trained. It is imperative that all staff be properly trained in the use of the advanced technology or new equipment.

Privileges for new skills (eg, laparoscopic morcellator, harmonic scalpel) should only be granted when the appropriate training has been completed and documented and the competency level has been achieved with adequate supervision. That is, each physician requesting additional privileges for new equipment or technology should be evaluated by answering the following questions:

   1. Does the hospital have a mechanism in place to ensure that necessary support for the new equipment or technology is available?

   2. Has the physician been adequately trained, including hands-on experience, to use the new equipment or to perform the new technology?

   3. Has the physician adequately demonstrated an ability to use the new equipment or perform the new technology? This may require that the physician undergo a period of proctoring or supervision, or both. If no one on staff can serve as a proctor, the hospital may either require reciprocal proctoring at another hospital or grant temporary privileges to someone from another hospital to supervise the applicant.

Specifically, if the new privileges were not included in residency training, the applicant must:

   1. Complete a preceptorship with a physician already credentialed to perform the procedures of that skill level; the preceptorship should require the applicant to perform the designated surgery with the preceptor acting as first-assistant.

   2. Provide a list of cases satisfactorily completed under supervision at each skill level, as defined by the local institution.

   3. Submit a letter from the preceptor documenting that the procedures were completed in a satisfactory manner and that the applicant is competent to perform the procedures independently at the designated skill level.

If there is no experienced surgeon on the hospital staff who is able to serve as a preceptor for advanced or new surgical procedures, a supervised preceptorship must be arranged. This may be done by scheduling a number of cases from physicians requiring credentialing and inviting a credentialed surgeon from another institution to serve as a surgical consultant.

After a Period of Inactivity

The American Medical Association (AMA) defines physician reentry as "a return to clinical practice in the discipline in which one has been trained and certified following an extended period of inactivity" (3). This section will not address inactivity that results from discipline or impairment.

There are several reasons why a physician might take a leave of absence from clinical practice, such as family leave (maternity and paternity leave and child care); personal health reasons; career dissatisfaction; alternate careers such as administration; military service; or humanitarian leave. Traditionally, women were more likely to experience career interruptions; however, recent research shows that younger cohorts of male physicians also take on multiple roles and express intentions to adjust their careers accordingly (3).

When physicians request reentry after a period of inactivity, a general guideline for evaluation would be to consider the physician as any other new applicant for privileges. This would include evaluation of the following:

1. Demonstration that a minimum number of hours of continuing medical education has been earned during the period of inactivity. It is also important to meet any board certification requirements (see Part 4) during the absence.

2. In accordance with the medical staff bylaws, supervision by a proctor appointed by the department chair for a minimum number and defined breadth of cases during the provisional period, evaluating and documenting proficiency.

3. A time-sensitive, focused review of cases as required by the departmental quality improvement committee may be completed as appropriate.

The area of skills assessment may prove challenging if the previous guidelines, number 2 and number 3, are not felt to be adequate. But, there are several options to consider:

1. Residency Training Programs

   Benefits: More locations are available, providing structured didactic programs, and implementing competency assessment. Participating in these programs can provide a source of manpower to help compensate for restricted residency work hours.

   Drawbacks: Many hospitals with residency programs have only a limited number of cases available for training. Reentry programs must not negatively affect the residency training program (ie, if someone is being brought into a reentry program in an institution that has a residency program, the Residency Review Committee must be notified with an explanation as to how it will not negatively affect the residents).

2. Simulation Centers

   Benefits: These centers can help supplement hands-on clinical experience and may be more geographically accessible. The use of simulation centers for reentry into practice is a new concept. This training may precede and supplement proctored clinical experience.

   Drawbacks: Currently there is a limited number of functioning simulation centers, though this number should continue to expand. Cost is another drawback.

3. Physician Reentry Program (PREP)

   Benefits: Well designed PREP systems should be consistent with the current continuum of medical education and meet the needs of the reentering physician.

   Drawbacks: Only a few PREP systems are offered nationally; thus, cost and location are considerable obstacles in utilizing these programs.

An underlying assumption is that physicians do not necessarily lose competence in all areas of practice with time. Competencies such as patient communication and professionalism may not decline. Therefore, a reentry program should target those areas where physicians are more likely to have lost relevant skills or knowledge, or where skills and knowledge need to be updated (4).

Finally, it is extremely important for physicians considering a leave of absence or major change in practice activities to think in advance about options should they wish to return. At a minimum, licensure and continuing medical education activities should be maintained. Working part-time during an absence helps to maintain a minimal amount of competency.

For more information on credentialing, privileging, and accreditation, please refer to Appendix G, "Report of the Presidential Task Force on Patient Safety in the Office Setting." Refer to Appendix F for a sample application for privileges.

References

1. Greeley H, Harrington L, Pybus BE, Sheff RA. Core privileges: a practical approach to development and implementation. Marblehead (MA): Opus Communications; 2001.

2. American Academy of Family Physicians, American College of Obstetricians and Gynecologists. AAFP-ACOG joint statement on cooperative practice and hospital privileges. Leawood (KS): AAFP; Washington, DC: ACOG; 1998.

3. Mark S, Gupta J. Reentry into clinical practice: challenges and strategies. JAMA 2002;288:1091–6.

4. American Medical Association. Report 6 of the Council on Medical Education (A-08): physician reentry. Chicago (IL): AMA; 2008. Available at: http://www.ama-assn.org/ama1/pub/upload/mm/377/cmerpt_6a-08.pdf. Retrieved June 24, 2009.

PART 4

Quality Improvement and Patient Safety in the Outpatient Setting

Most information about patient safety and quality improvement (QI) has been written with respect to the hospital setting; however, it is only in recent years that this focus has expanded to include care provided in the outpatient setting. Experts are beginning to understand the nature of medical errors and how they occur in these clinical domains. Care provided in the outpatient setting is viewed as broader and often perceived as fragmented. Proficiency and expertise in the inpatient setting may not translate to the same level of care in the outpatient setting (1). Quality improvement in the outpatient setting presents unique challenges because 1) there is a much less formal mechanism for this type of review, 2) outpatient care is less structured than its inpatient counterpart, and 3) there is less oversight from a regulatory and legal perspective.

Although various sets of quality measures exist for care provided in the outpatient setting, the Healthcare Effectiveness Data and Information Set (HEDIS), developed by the National Committee for Quality Assurance (NCQA), is the most widely used. More than 90% of U.S. health plans use HEDIS measures to evaluate performance in important dimensions of care and service. Most HEDIS effectiveness-of-care measures evaluate care that is provided in outpatient settings. Although HEDIS data are gathered based on activities occurring at the individual physician level, the data are aggregated for analysis and recommendations by health plans.

Quality improvement efforts depend significantly on physician support; thus, physician leadership is crucial to the success of the quality movement (2, 3). Currently, this involvement and leadership needs to be strengthened. In a 2003 survey, only 34% of physicians had been involved in a redesign effort to improve patient care at either their offices or hospitals, and only 33% had access to any type of quality data (4). In a study of small practices (five or fewer physicians) working with a state Quality Improvement Organization, most physicians had never received training in QI principles and methods, and definitions of QI varied widely among physicians (5). This lack of understanding among providers in small office settings proved to be a significant barrier. Office staff also lacked understanding and skills related to QI, another critical barrier to bringing about improvement.

In a study of what drives QI in small to moderate practices, the American Board of Internal Medicine Foundation and the National Committee for Quality Assurance found that motivation was the most important factor that determined participation and development in QI projects (6). The impetus for change occurred when an internal leader (refer to the section "Physician Champions" in Part 2) was presented data that indicated suboptimal care was being provided by the practice. Most physicians believed they were giving the best care, but when shown otherwise, internal motivation led them to develop and participate in strategies for improvement.

There are many reasons for limited physician involvement in QI activities. They may stem from a lack of exposure to QI movement literature and the perception that participation in the movement requires sophisticated information technology systems, access to a large database, multiple resources for the collection and analysis of data, and expensive systems for ongoing monitoring.

Collection of data may be accomplished by internally driven organizational mandates, or requirements may be imposed by external sources. If a practice or plan finds it necessary to meet several different reporting requirements and QI priorities from varying external sources, meeting these needs may draw attention and resources away from patient care or internal QI efforts. In recognition of this, numerous expert panels have commented on the need for greater standardization of reporting requirements for performance measurement (7, 8).

Since 2004, the AQA (originally known as the Ambulatory Care Quality Alliance), a broad-based group of physicians, consumers, purchasers, health insurance plans, and others, has been collaborating on performance measurement, data aggregation, and reporting in the ambulatory setting (9). Concurrent with this effort is an increasing interest in the development of a reimbursement system that offers incentives for quality health care (ie, pay for performance). It is clear that demands for better measures of quality in ambulatory care will only increase.

Challenges of Developing a Performance Measurement System

There are a number of challenges to developing a performance measurement framework for physician organizations. Listed are questions to consider at the beginning of the development process (10):

- What will be the specific purposes of the measurement system?

- How should the specific aspects of performance for which individual physicians or physician organizations will be held accountable be measured?

- What specific information should be part of the performance measurement system and included in the reporting system? What are the optimal formats for disseminating performance information?

- How will performance measures for physicians or physician organizations be implemented in an ongoing and feasibly sustainable way? Who will bear its costs?

Meaningful reporting at the practice level is a challenge. For example, the challenges for measuring performance in small practices include lack of infrastructure, lack of health information technology, lack of support staff, and increased burden of data collection (11). A 2003 survey found that less than one fourth of physicians had the ability to compare their performance with their peers either within their specialty or within health plans (12). Only 11% had the capacity to meet the benchmark of physicians nationally (12).

Public and private purchaser data must be pooled to yield meaningful information on small practice settings. Individual insurers do not account for a large enough share of a practice's population to provide meaningful measures of performance. Some aspects of practice performance are quite difficult to assess; this is particularly true if a practitioner sees a low volume of patients, in which case there will not be enough data to provide meaningful or valid assessments of performance. When sample sizes are small, there are problems with risk adjustment and bias, and although these issues may be dealt with, there is currently no mechanism for pooling data across purchasers (13). Whereas all providers involved in the care of a patient share in the responsibility for providing quality care, designing measurement systems that accurately reflect the degree of influence and responsibility of each practitioner is problematic at best (14). Principles for using measurement to support improvement in the busy, ambulatory setting are listed in Box 4-1 (15). Box 2-1 and Box 2-2 in Part 2 also may be useful in guiding performance improvement activities in the outpatient setting.

Peer Review

Peer review is "the critical evaluation of a specific aspect of a practitioner's performance by professional colleagues, preferably achieved through use of a reliable and structured instrument" (16, 17). Peer review should be used as a learning tool to provide feedback on physician performance, not a disciplinary action.

Conducting peer review in the outpatient and office setting is challenging, particularly because of limited external oversight. The Joint Commission and the Accreditation Association for Ambulatory Health Care (AAAHC) have accreditation programs for ambulatory care and office-based surgery. The Joint Commission requires a "process that defines circumstances requiring a focused review of a practitioner's performance and evaluation of a practitioner's performance by peers" (18). The Joint Commission stipulates the elements of a focused review process, but gives latitude by simply requiring, for example, that the process identify the circumstances under which external peer review is conducted.

The Accreditation Association for Ambulatory Health Care accreditation standards for ambulatory health care

---

Box 4-1. Principles for Using Measurement to Support Improvement in Busy Ambulatory Settings

- Seek relevance in the measurement

- Use a balanced set of process, outcome, and cost measures

- Keep measurements simple (focus on a manageable set of measures). Use measures that are applicable to large numbers of patients or that have baseline performance rates in the range of 40–60%

- Use both qualitative and quantitative data (quantitative data measures need for change and impact of changes, whereas qualitative data measures how people feel about the need or impact of the changes)

- Clearly define, in writing, the operational definitions of each measure (provide a clear method for scoring or measuring each variable so measurement collection is easily reproducible)

- Measure small but representative samples (it is not necessary to measure every patient all of the time)

- Build measurements into the daily flow of work (make scoring and measurement easy)

- Develop a measurement team (share the load and build camaraderie in the endeavor)

Nelson EC, Splaine ME, Batalden PB, Plume SK. Building measurement and data collection into medical practice. Ann Intern Med 1998;128:460–6.

require that "an accreditable organization maintains an active and organized process for peer review that is integrated into the quality management and improvement program" (19). The standards require at least two physicians to be involved to provide peer-based review, but require an outside physician to be involved to provide peer-based review in solo physician organizations.

Few individual office practices are accredited by either of these organizations, which leave individual physicians with complete responsibility for the quality and safety of patient care provided under their purview. However, maintenance of certification offers a mechanism for sustaining professionalism and instituting quality improvement.

Maintenance of Certification

Evaluation of the structural elements in systems that affect quality and the ability to aggregate and evaluate physicians at the group, health plan, and hospital levels has improved. Reliable and valid clinical performance assessment of individual physicians, however, will require a great deal more research and development. Many believe that the traditional measure of physician quality—certification—is an adequate measure of quality alone. Certification by a medical specialty board is meant to indicate that a physician has the knowledge, skill, and competency to provide quality care.

As mandated by the American Board of Medical Specialties (ABMS), all medical specialty boards now require physicians with time-limited certification to participate in a Maintenance of Certification (MOC) program. Between 2000 and 2006, all of the major medical specialties began developing programs that require these physicians to continually update their certification through MOC. All specialty boards are currently implementing their respective ABMS-approved MOC programs. This was done, in part, as a response to demands for ongoing quality monitoring of physicians and the health care system and the belief that certification programs are adequate and sufficient measures of knowledge and competence (20).

Maintenance of Certification calls for evidence of 1) professional standing, 2) lifelong learning and periodic assessment, 3) cognitive expertise as demonstrated by a secure examination, and 4) performance in practice. All 24 specialty boards that are members of the ABMS have agreed to design methods to meet these requirements (20). In 2003, the ABMS encouraged its member boards to introduce the subject of patient safety in their respective certification and MOC examinations. To address questions surrounding this decision, ABMS and the Council of Medical Specialty Societies convened a panel of patient safety experts. The panel created a list of areas eligible for inclusion in upcoming examinations: epidemiology of medical error and harm, general meth-

odology of patient safety, specific systems factors, and safety practices. Boards may test on how errors occur in medical care, how they could be prevented, and what to do when errors occur. Questions related to the physician's ethical and legal obligations to the patient after an error has occurred are permissible (21).

Maintenance of Certification from the American Board of Obstetrics and Gynecology

Beginning in 2001, all new certificates issued by the American Board of Obstetrics and Gynecology (ABOG) were 6 years in duration. Beginning in 2008, all newly board-certified obstetrician–gynecologists automatically began the annual MOC process. In addition, as the certifications expire for those physicians with time-limited certification, they too will begin MOC.

Methods for Maintenance of Certification

Voluntary Recertification

Voluntary recertification applies only to those diplomates whose certification occurred prior to 1986 (in general obstetrics and gynecology) or 1987 (in the subspecialties). These individuals have no time limitation on their certificates. Not participating in MOC will not have an impact on their board certification. Even though ABOG does not require these physicians to participate in MOC, at some point their states or hospitals may eventually require them to participate.

Certificate Renewal

Certificate renewal, an option between 1986 and 1987 and the implementation of MOC, is no longer available. Certificate renewal applies to diplomates with time-limited certificates (certificates issued in or after 1986 for general obstetrician–gynecologists and in or after 1987 for subspecialists). The time granted for each method is listed as follows. Both voluntary recertification and certificate renewal could be obtained by one of three methods:

1. Written examination: 6 years' duration
2. Oral examination: 6 years' duration
3. Annual board certification: annual certification plus at least 25 Continuing Medical Education credits

Annual Maintenance of Certification

All newly board-certified ob-gyns and physicians with time-limited certificates are required to participate in MOC to continue ABOG certification. Maintenance of certification is a four-part program to be completed over each 6-year MOC cycle:

> Part 1: ABOG reviews the physician's license annually
>
> Part 2: Annual article reviews and questions

Part 3: A written examination. The examination will be offered for the first time in 2012. Each physician must complete the examination by the end of the 6-year MOC cycle.

Part 4: Complete 10 self-assessment modules by the end of the 6-year MOC cycle

For additional information regarding annual maintenance of certification, go to www.acog.org/from_home/Misc/mocReminder.cfm.

Maintenance of Certification is a potentially meaningful measure of competency, but there is not a strong base of evidence to conclude this. The development of measures of quality that truly and fully reflect the higher level of decision making skills and care required of physicians remains to be done. The impact of MOC interventions to promote QI remains ill-defined, a point that should be kept in mind as there is some discussion about the use of MOC activities to be used in pay-for-performance programs.

Elements of a Patient Safety Program in the Outpatient Setting

Although most outpatient care is delivered in the physician's office, care also may be provided in other settings such as surgery centers, emergency rooms, occupational and mental health centers, and diagnostic imaging centers. As more attention is directed toward patient safety in the outpatient setting, focus must be placed on how health care providers communicate with patients. Physicians must partner with patients to manage and direct their care by providing information in a format that takes into account the patients' health literacy and willingness and ability to participate in their care. Systems that document and track how care is rendered and facilitate improved communication among all health care providers are essential for improving care over the continuum.

Communication and Patient Health Literacy

When communication breaks down, patients are at risk. The factors that contribute to communication failure are widespread and include system and health care provider performance issues. These factors may include delays in care, failure to follow up on abnormal results due to workload, and failure to establish a system for tracking. It also may be difficult to obtain all available patient history and results, particularly when multiple health care providers from different systems are involved in a patient's care. The absence of back-up systems to ensure proper communication, that is, planned redundancy, can be very expensive, and human error due to missed and delayed diagnoses, fatigue, health care provider

workload, interruptions, and multiple handoffs all place patients at increased risk (22, 23).

The Institute of Medicine defines health literacy as "the degree to which individuals have the capacity to obtain, process, and understand basic health information and services needed to make appropriate health decisions" (24). Patients must be able to understand the information given to them and then translate that into appropriate actions to adhere to prescribed medical advice. Health literacy is an issue of understanding rather than of access to medical information. Those especially at risk are elderly individuals, recent immigrants, individuals with chronic disease, and those of low socioeconomic status (24, 25). Many organizations, including the Institute of Medicine, U.S. Department of Health and Human Services, American Medical Association, Harvard School of Public Health, and the Agency for Healthcare Research and Quality, have published information and made recommendations for improving patient safety by providing tools and educational materials for practitioners.

Low health literacy affects millions of U.S. adults, and this can cause serious consequences to the individuals and to the system as a whole. Low health literacy is associated with adverse health outcomes, increased health care costs, and increased emergency room visits. In 1998, the National Academy on an Aging Society estimated that the inability to understand medical directions cost more than $73 billion in additional health care costs (26). Literacy skills are a stronger predictor of a person's health status than age, income, employment status, education level, and racial or ethnic group. Improving clear health communication is everyone's responsibility (27). Poor health literacy is a silent epidemic, one that can be difficult to identify because many patients have developed various coping strategies. For example, patients may give written material to a partner or family member with them, or say "I'll read this at home." Patients also may respond by being aloof or withdrawn while a health care provider discusses their care.

Many public and private organizations continue to raise awareness, publish information, maintain web sites, and develop patient education materials for improving patient safety and providing tools for practitioners and patients to improve communication and understanding. For the practitioner, examples include the Newest Vital Sign developed by Pfizer to assess general literacy and numeracy skills as applied to health information, yielding an overall assessment of health literacy, and Pfizer's *Principles for Clear Health Communication Handbook* to educate and assist practitioners in their encounters with patients to ensure better patient understanding (28). For patients, there are also online videos by organizations such as the American Medical Association and the Harvard School of Public Health to raise awareness and stimulate discussion about health literacy. There are also many web sites dedicated to assisting in developing and writing patient education materials to include readability formulas and health clip-art, graphics, and illustrations to communicate important information about the patient's condition and how to follow recommended treatments. Most patients forget 80% of what a health care provider tells them as soon as they leave the office, and 50% of what they do recall is recalled incorrectly (28). There are techniques the practitioner can use to improve retention and understanding of important information, such as the "teach-back" method, where the patient repeats her understanding of the information back to the practitioner. Providing visual aids or using other tools may help increase the amount of information retained by patients. Becoming an active listener by encouraging patients to talk is also helpful.

Other techniques include avoidance of acronyms and words with multiple meanings, being aware of and addressing quizzical looks, and taking a pause to slow down the encounter. All these techniques and resources can be used to create a welcoming and supportive environment that can improve communication and ensure patient understanding.

Partnering With Patients

The Institute for Family-Centered Care, in collaboration with the Institute for Healthcare Improvement, began to explore how to enhance collaboration with patients and families and realize the enormous potential of patient and family partnerships. A roadmap was created to design the patient and family health care system for the future. A work in progress, the history of patient- and family-centered care is discussed as follows.

To understand what partnering with patients means in health care, an understanding of the key concept of patient- and family-centered care is important. This term was first introduced in 1969 by Michael Balint as "patient-centered medicine" (29). The Picker Institute then coined the term "patient-centered care" in 1988 in an effort to understand the patient's definition of high quality care. In the United States, Canada, and Europe, patient experiences were measured in eight dimensions:

1. Access
2. Respect for patient values and preferences
3. Coordination of care
4. Information, communication, and education
5. Physical comfort
6. Emotional support
7. Involvement of friends and family
8. Preparation for discharge and transitions in care

These are deemed the most critical aspects of the care experienced by patients and their families (29).

The 1960s and 1970s saw a family-centered care evolution in maternity services. Parents of children dependent on technological support sought to work in a more collaborative manner with health care professionals and successfully advocated for legislation that would enable them to care for their children in home and community settings. U.S. Surgeon General C. Everett Koop, along with leaders in organizations such as the Maternal and Child Health Bureau of the U.S. Department of Health and Human Services and the Association for the Care of Children's Health, advanced the practice of family-centered care by focusing on children with special health care needs, and by the end of the 1980s, these leaders collaborated with women and families affected by HIV infection and AIDS to apply similar systems. Recently, patient- and family-centered care have evolved to link this perspective with the concept of collaboration in planning, implementing, and evaluating systems of care for patients of all ages, at all levels of care, and in all health care settings (30). This concept recognizes that the very young, the very old, and those with chronic conditions are most dependent on the health care system and also most dependent on their families. Family members are essential members of the caregiving team (29).

According to the Institute for Family-Centered Care, there are four core concepts of patient- and family-centered care (29):

1. Dignity and respect—Providers honor patient and family perspective and choices, and patient and family knowledge, values, beliefs, and culture are incorporated into the care.
2. Information sharing—Patients and families need timely, complete, and accurate information in order to effectively participate in care and decision making.
3. Participation—Patients and families are encouraged to participate at whatever level they choose.
4. Collaboration—Providers and patients collaborate in planning, implementing, and evaluating systems of care.

In order to adapt these concepts, cultural change is needed. Health care providers need to believe that patient participation is essential to the design and delivery of optimal care. This would then help redesign health care safety and quality, leading to better outcomes and a more gratifying, creative, and inspiring way to practice (31).

Strategies aimed at implementing patient- and family-centered care are becoming available as the momentum for change in the outpatient setting is critical in optimizing individual and family health. These strategies include developing and supporting partnerships among administrators, health care providers, patients, and families to improve quality and safety in ambulatory care. Having families, administrators, and health care providers on the same team is valuable in making decisions about facilities, activities, and the clinical encounter itself. To ensure that these processes continue and are followed through, it is essential to have a framework for appropriate interventions.

Medication Safety

As in the inpatient setting, medication safety is the number one quality concern in the outpatient setting. The National Center for Health Statistics reported that clinicians wrote approximately 2 billion prescriptions in 2005. Medications were "provided, prescribed, or continued" at 70.5% of all office visits. A 2003 study concluded that adverse events related to medications are common, and many are preventable (32). In this prospective study, which included a survey of patients and a chart review, 162 of the 661 patients responding had an adverse drug event (25%). Twenty-four of these events (13%) were classified as serious, 51 (28%) were ameliorable, and 20 (11%) were preventable. Of the 51 ameliorable events, 32 (63%) were attributed to the physician's failure to respond to medication-related symptoms and 19 (37%) were attributed to the patient's failure to inform the physician of the symptoms. In addition, the Massachusetts State Board of Registration in Pharmacy has estimated that 2.4 million prescriptions are filled improperly each year, and 90% are filled improperly because of the wrong drug or dosage. These errors are commonly attributed to inadequate point of care access to current clinical knowledge or unavailable patient data (33).

Fewer protections and safeguards are available in the outpatient setting than in the inpatient setting. There is often a lack of protocols and standardization to ensure correct drug name, dose, route, and time. A major difference in the outpatient versus the inpatient setting is the increased role of patients and families in providing care as well as the multiple sites of care. Clinicians must seek opportunities for partnering with patients in medication safety. Partnering with patients will improve patient satisfaction and reduce opportunities for error. Clear, simplified communication is essential. The physician should provide information and instruction through various mediums, including verbal, written, and audiovisual, and make certain the patient knows what each drug is for, the potential side effects, and the signs of serious side effects that would warrant her immediately calling the physician. Encourage patients to carry a current medication list, and do not assume that all health care providers have shared information. Check on patients' medications and have them "teach-back" their routine with brown bag prescription bottle checks by having them bring all their prescriptions in a bag and having them explain why they take them. Be sure to communicate with other members of the health care team, such as the patient's preferred pharmacist, and know what other health care providers the patient has seen since her last visit. Finally, collaborate with nursing and other office staff to streamline and coordinate information during each office visit.

Tracking and Reminder Systems

Tracking and reminder systems play a key role in the assurance of quality care and patient safety. Current systems are inefficient, and there are many opportunities for failure to follow-up. The challenge is to keep tracking systems simple and accessible for ongoing updating and monitoring (23).

There is an enormous burden on the health care provider to manage the results of outpatient tests. Research has shown that the average time spent managing test results per clinic day was approximately 72 minutes, and when surveyed, 41% of physicians responded not being satisfied with the way they managed test results (34). Failure to follow up may lead to a missed or a delayed diagnosis, which may result in adverse patient outcome or potential liability for the health care provider. One study showed that one half of missed diagnoses due to failure to follow up involved a cancer diagnosis, primarily breast and colorectal. No other diagnosis accounted for more than 5% of the sample in this study. Most of these breakdowns involved many factors both by the practitioner and the patient, with most linked to a single-point breakdown (35). The resultant delays are long, sometimes delaying the diagnosis for more than a year. Much attention has been given to the development of tracking systems in order to keep health care providers and patients on track with their care. These systems and tools need to be automated and easy to use in order to be integrated into the health care provider's work flow.

For the obstetrician–gynecologist, tracking systems can be individualized and prioritized to the office needs. Common tracking needs include cervical cytology results and appropriate follow-up; need for colposcopy; mammogram and follow-up; laboratory tests; radiology studies; pathology reports; routine and specific obstetric testing such as sequential screening and antenatal testing; after hours and on-call emergencies from covering health care providers, hospitals, and emergency departments; follow-up appointments; and specialty referrals. Once an established protocol is formed, whether manual or electronic, the entire process from data entry through reconciliation needs to be reviewed on an ongoing basis to ensure its effectiveness. Encouraging all personnel who participate in tracking patients' care to provide input into the system's development will encourage its use and decrease the risk of system failure. Ease of use and standardization should be emphasized, and responsibility should not rest on one person (23).

The challenges to a well-designed tracking system include patient failure to comply with follow-up plans;

coordination of care, including specialty referrals, among the potentially high volume of outpatient tests and procedures; multiple care locations; and fragmentation of care, leading to an "out of sight, out of mind" mindset. Increased expectations by patients of their health care providers and the health care system for such things as early diagnosis of cancer and timely communication of test results also pose significant challenges.

In one study, poor patient adherence to follow-up plans accounted for 56% (45 of 81) of errors that contributed to poor outcome. This emphasizes the need for risk-reduction interventions that address both sides of the health care provider–patient relationship during follow-up (32). The process of good patient follow-up begins at the initial visit with the practitioner explaining to the patient the benefits of any tests or referrals, ensuring that the patient understands their importance. The follow-up recommendations, tests, and referrals should be logged into a system that will be regularly reviewed based on established office protocols.

Coordination of care among multiple health care providers is a priority that the Joint Commission has addressed in its National Patient Safety Goal 2, "improve the effectiveness of communication among caregivers." Although this goal was intended primarily for verbal communication within the hospital system, it also should address the gaps in communication in the outpatient setting, where information can easily fall through the cracks. Often, breakdowns in follow-up occur because of unclear definitions of adequate follow-up and lack of communication strategies and backup or automated mechanisms to allow delivery of information. In addition, with multiple health care providers giving care, there may be no specific delineation of responsibility. For example, confusion may arise if the requisition is incomplete or the ordering health care provider is not the health care provider who performs the follow-up. Another concern is what should be done if the ordering health care provider cannot be reached by page or phone.

The transition from hospital care to outpatient care is another potential problematic area, especially when relaying test results that may be pending at discharge. A recent study of two tertiary care hospital systems found that physicians were unaware of abnormal and potentially actionable post-discharge test results more than 60% of the time (36). This demonstrates the importance of establishing clear responsibilities and developing tools to keep track of pending test results at discharge and communicating those results to outpatient health care providers. It also emphasizes the importance of the discharge summary as an important document where all pending tests and follow-up plans should be detailed.

Information technologies that are integrated into the electronic medical record, identify abnormal test results, generate appropriate reminders, and incorporate evidence-based guidelines to assist health care provid-ers can aid in minimizing variability and fragmentation and improve quality and safety in the outpatient setting. Health care providers' comfort with information technology systems may vary. Ongoing training as well as continued support is necessary for successful implementation of these strategies.

References

1. Wachter RM. Is ambulatory patient safety just like hospital safety, only without the "stat"? Ann Intern Med 2006;145:547–9.

2. Brennan TA. Physicians' professional responsibility to improve the quality of care. Acad Med 2002;77:973–80.

3. Bradley EH, Holmboe ES, Mattera JA, Roumanis SA, Radford MJ, Krumholz HM. A qualitative study of increasing beta-blocker use after myocardial infarction: why do some hospitals succeed? JAMA 2001;285:2604–11.

4. Audet AM, Doty MM, Shamasdin J, Schoenbaum SC. Measure, learn, and improve: physicians' involvement in quality improvement. Health Aff 2005;24:843–53.

5. Holmboe E, Kim N, Cohen S, Curry M, Elwell A, Petrillo MK, et al. Health care physicians, office-based practice, and the meaning of quality improvement. Am J Med 2005;118:917–22.

6. Wolfson D, Bernabeo E, Leas B, Sofaer S, Pawlson G, Pillittere D. Quality improvement in small office settings: an examination of successful practices. BMC Fam Pract 2009;10:14.

7. Institute of Medicine (US). The future of the public's health in the 21st century. Washington, DC: National Academies Press; 2003.

8. President's Advisory Commission on Consumer Protection and Quality in the Health Care Industry. Quality first: better health care for all Americans. Bethesda (MD): PACCPQHCI; 1998. http://www.hcqualitycommission.gov/final. Retrieved June 24, 2009.

9. Agency for Healthcare Research and Quality. The Ambulatory Care Quality Alliance recommended starter set: clinical performance measures for ambulatory care. Rockville (MD): AHRQ; 2005. Available at: http://www.ahrq.gov/qual/aqastart.pdf. Retrieved June 17, 2009.

10. Roski J, Gregory R. Performance measurement for ambulatory care: moving towards a new agenda. Int J Qual Health Care 2001;13:447–53.

11. Landon BE, Normand SL. Performance measurement in the small office practice: challenges and potential solutions. Ann Intern Med 2008;148:353–7.

12. Audet AM, Doty MM, Shamasdin J, Schoenbaum SC. Physicians' views on quality of care: findings from the Commonwealth Fund National Survey of Physicians and Quality of Care. New York (NY): Commonwealth Fund; 2005. Available at: http://www.commonwealthfund.org/usr_doc/823Audet_physiciansurveychartpack.pdf. Retrieved June 17, 2009.

13. Milstein A. Hot potato endgame. Health Aff 2004;23:32–4.

14. Institute of Medicine (US). Performance measurement: accelerating improvement. Washington, DC: National Academies Press; 2006.

15. Nelson EC, Splaine ME, Batalden PB, Plume SK. Building measurement and data collection into medical practice. Ann Intern Med 1998;128:460–6.

16. Norcini JJ. Peer assessment of competence. Med Educ 2003; 37:539–43.

17. Grol R. Quality improvement by peer review in primary care: a practical guide. Qual Health Care 1994;3:147–52.

18. The Joint Commission. There is a process that defines circumstances requiring a focused review of a practitioner's performance and evaluation of a practitioner's performance by peers. Standard HR.4.34. In: Comprehensive accreditation manual for ambulatory care. Oakbrook Terrace (IL): Joint Commission; 2008. p. HR-15–HR-16.

19. Accreditation Association for Ambulatory Health Care. Subchapter I—peer review. In: Accreditation handbook for ambulatory health care. Skokie (IL): AAAHC; 2008. p. 30–1.

20. Brennan TA, Horwitz RI, Duffy FD, Cassel CK, Goode LD, Lipner RS. The role of physician specialty board certification status in the quality movement. JAMA 2004;292: 1038–43.

21. Kachalia A, Johnson JK, Miller S, Brennan T. The incorporation of patient safety into board certification examinations. Acad Med 2006;81:317–25.

22. Gandhi TK. Fumbled handoffs: one dropped ball after another. Ann Intern Med 2005;142:352–8.

23. Tracking and reminder systems. ACOG Committee Opinion No. 329. American College of Obstetricians and Gynecologists. Obstet Gynecol 2006;107:745–7.

24. Institute of Medicine (US). Health literacy: a prescription to end confusion. Washington, DC: National Academies Press; 2004.

25. Health literacy. ACOG Committee Opinion No. 391. American College of Obstetricians and Gynecologists. Obstet Gynecol 2007;110:1489–91.

26. VA Library Network. Health literacy resources. Available at: http://www.mdmlg.org/Health-Literacy-Resources.pdf. Retrieved June 17, 2009.

27. National Patient Safety Foundation. Eradicating low health literacy: the first public health movement of the 21st century. Boston (MA): NPSF; 2003. Available at: http://www.npsf.org/askme3/pdfs/white_paper.pdf. Retrieved June 17, 2009.

28. Pfizer. Pfizer clear health communication initiative. Available at: http://www.pfizerhealthliteracy.com. Retrieved June 17, 2009.

29. Institute for Family-Centered Care. Partnering with patients and families to design a patient- and family-centered health care system: a roadmap for the future: a work in progress. Bethesda (MD): IFCC; 2006. Available at: http://www.familycenteredcare.org/pdf/Roadmap.pdf. Retrieved June 17, 2009.

30. Institute for Family Centered Care, Institute for Healthcare Improvement. Partnering with patients and families to design a patient- and family-centered health care system: recommendations and promising practices. Bethesda (MD): IFCC; Cambridge (MA): IHI; 2008.

31. Partnering with patients to improve safety. ACOG Committee Opinion No. 320. American College of Obstetricians and Gynecologists. Obstet Gynecol 2005;106:1123–5.

32. Gandhi TK, Weingart SN, Borus J, Seger AC, Peterson J, Burdick E, et al. Patient Safety: adverse drug events in ambulatory care. N Engl J Med 2003;348:1556–64.

33. National Patient Safety Foundation. Collaborative leadership for patient safety for ambulatory surgery in the office setting: phase I report of the National Patient Safety Consensus for the Community of Stakeholders for Ambulatory Surgery in the Office Setting. Boston (MA): NPSF; 2002. Available at: http://www.npsf.org/download/ASOSFinalReport.pdf. Retrieved June 18, 2009.

34. Poon EG, Gandhi TK, Sequist TD, Murff HJ, Karson AS, Bates DW. "I wish I had seen this test result earlier!": dissatisfaction with test result management systems in primary care. Arch Intern Med 2004;164:2223–8.

35. Gandhi TK, Kachalia A, Thomas EJ, Puopolo AL, Yoon C, Brennan TA, et al. Missed and delayed diagnoses in the ambulatory setting: a study of closed malpractice claims. Ann Intern Med 2006;145:488–96.

36. Roy CL, Poon EG, Karson AS, Ladak-Merchant Z, Johnson RE, Maviglia SM, et al. Patient safety concerns arising from test results that return after hospital discharge. Ann Intern Med 2005;143:121–8.

PART 5

Tools

Various tools for data analysis and quality measurement are used to identify, examine, improve, or change health care provision processes. These tools allow health care providers to target problems areas, track performance, and develop strategies to ensure quality and safety in health care delivery.

Data Analysis Tools

In order to improve the quality of health care, it is important to first identify the nature of the problem to be addressed. This in turn requires the collection of data regarding processes of care and an understanding of the nature and cause of statistical variation in those data. Tools are necessary to apply to those data to embark on a quality improvement path that converts raw data into useful information, information into knowledge about processes of care, and finally, knowledge into correct and wise actions. Data analysis tools help 1) identify the process that needs improvement, 2) identify the part of the process that needs improvement, and 3) assess the results of proposed intervention (1).

Variation is inherent in any system or process in the natural world. This completely random type of variation is called "common cause" variation. If a system or process is subject only to common cause variation, a graph of the frequency of given values results in a pattern we instantly recognize as a classic bell-shaped curve. In an ideal bell-shaped curve, the mean, median, and mode are all identical. The mean is the average of all values, the median is the value at which one half of all results lie above and one half below, and the mode is the value with the greatest frequency. However, even "ideal" bell-shaped curves do not all look alike—some are tall and narrow, and some are low and broad. The mathematical term to describe these differences is "standard deviation" (SD). It is a measure of the difference of values in the curve from the mean; curves with high standard deviation are broad and those with low standard deviation are narrow. An interesting characteristic of all bell-shaped curves related to standard deviation is the so-called

"68–95–99.7 rule." Sixty-eight percent of results will fall within 1 SD of the mean, 95% within 2 SD of the mean, and 99.7% within 3 SD of the mean. Generally, one of the goals in quality improvement is to reduce variability in outcomes, which can be thought of in statistical terms as creating a tall, narrow bell-shaped curve of results with a very small SD.

A second important type of variation is called "special cause" variation. This is a nonrandom, irregular change or event in a process that graphically appears as a "spike" or disruption in a smooth, symmetrical bell-shaped curve (Fig. 5-1). This type of variation is not inherent in the process or system itself. In quality improvement, it is often critical to distinguish between common cause and special cause variation because the approach to improving outcomes will be very different in each case (2).

If only common cause variation is present in a process, that process is spoken of as being "in control." If in addition to common cause variation there is special cause variation present, that process is spoken of as being "out of control." If a process is out of control (ie, special cause variation is present and causing poor outcomes), then the solution will involve eliminating this special cause. If a process is in control (ie, special cause variation is absent), but the process is just not achieving the desired result, then improvement will require a redesign of part, or all, of the process. The tools described as follows help distinguish between these two types of variation.

Run Chart

A run chart is a graphic record of the outcomes of a process over time. The y-axis represents the units of the outcome being measured, and the x-axis represents whatever units are the appropriate intervals for the process being evaluated. A run chart requires an initial data set of 15–20 points that are plotted on the graph (Fig. 5-2). A median line is then drawn parallel to the x-axis that evenly divides the points above and below, and then a second line is used to connect each point. After each interval going forward, a new point is added to the chart

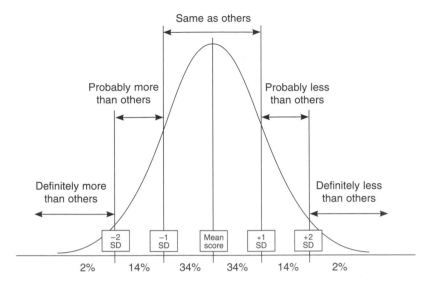

Fig. 5-1. Sample Bell-Shaped Curve.

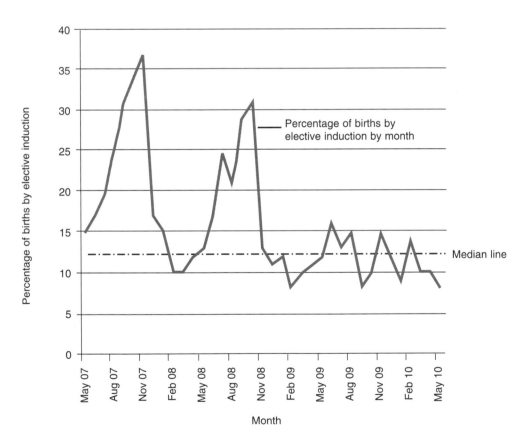

Fig. 5-2. Example of a Run Chart.

and the data line is extended. Common cause variation will cause the data line to move back and forth across the median. If special cause variation is present, there will be 8 or more data points on the same side of the median line, 6 or more points that steadily increase or decrease, or 14 points that alternately go up and down.

Control Chart

A control chart is a special category of run chart. A control chart is constructed similarly to a run chart, but the center line is the mean of all values (as opposed to the median in a run chart), and two additional lines parallel to the x-axis are added (Fig. 5-3). One above the center line is called the "upper control limit" and one below the center line is called the "lower control limit." These are calculated to correspond to 3 SD from the mean value. As we know from the previous discussion, this means that 99.7% of all values will fall between the two control limits if the process is in control. Therefore, if special cause variation

is present, this will be signaled by any of the conditions previously listed for run charts. In addition, even a single data point above or below the control limits indicates that a special cause of variation is present.

Histogram

Another useful tool for looking at process performance is a histogram. This is a special type of bar graph used to look at a single large set of process outcomes. It is especially useful for continuous variables such as time, weight, size, or temperature. The continuous variable data are divided into 10–12 groups of equal interval along the horizontal axis, and vertical bars reflect the frequency of results within each interval. The bars are then plotted on a graph with the x-axis being the outcome variable and the y-axis being frequency of result. The bars are placed directly adjacent to each other (Fig. 5-4), unless there are one or more intervals with a frequency of zero. If a process is in control, the results bar graph

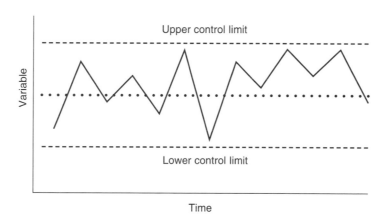

Fig. 5-3. Example of a Control Chart.

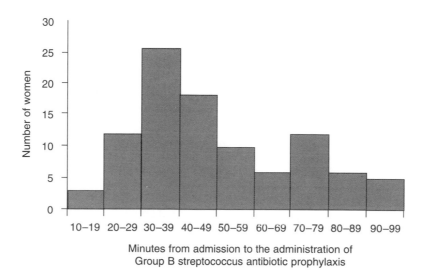

Fig. 5-4. Example of a Histogram.

will closely resemble a bell-shaped curve. Other shapes, such as long tails, double peaks, plateaus, or outlier peaks often can give useful insight as to how a process can be improved. For example, the histogram in Figure 5-4 depicts a lag time between admission of patients to a labor and delivery suite and the administration of Group B streptococcus antibiotic prophylaxis. Rather than a bell-shaped curve, there is a suggestion of a first peak at 30–39 minutes and a second peak around 70–79 minutes. This suggests that those patients on the right hand end of the curve should be evaluated to see why their antibiotic administration is being delayed.

Identifying a process that needs to be improved will facilitate focusing on where to direct improvement efforts. Processes to measure might include high-volume, high-risk, problem-prone procedures; resource intensive processes; sentinel events; and those outlined in the Joint Commission's National Patient Safety Goals. The following tools help identify what specific steps in a process need to be altered to produce the most improvement in outcomes.

Cause and Effect Diagram

A cause and effect diagram, also called a "fishbone diagram" or "Ishikawa diagram," is used to identify possible causes of a poor outcome. Typically, the poor outcome being investigated is identified in a box to the far right of the diagram, with a straight line drawn from the left. This represents the "head" and "spine" of a fish for which the diagram is named. From the spine are drawn several diagonal lines extending to the left, representing broad categories where problems may occur. These can be customized to the situation, but typical ones used in the health care setting are people, environment, equipment, materials, machinery, policies, and procedures. Using these major divisions, a process improvement team would brainstorm all possible causes for the poor out-

come, which are then depicted as short lines parallel to the spine coming off the diagonal "bones." Sometimes, given causes are further subdivided into additional contributing factors. When completed, a diagram of this type will help the team identify possible targets for process improvement efforts. The fishbone diagram (Fig. 5-5) is often used in performing a root cause analysis to retrospectively determine the causes of an adverse outcome. It also can be prospectively used in a Failure Mode and Effects Analysis to determine potential vulnerabilities in a process before there is an adverse outcome. The potential shortcoming of the fishbone analysis is neglecting to include all of the broad areas (bones) that may be relevant.

Pareto Chart

After several potential causes for poor outcome are identified, a Pareto chart (Fig. 5-6) can be used to determine which of many possible causes should be addressed first. It is named after Vilfredo Pareto, a 19th–century Italian economist who determined that 80% of the wealth of his nation was controlled by only 20% of the population. This so-called "80–20" rule became known as the Pareto principle and has found wide application in many fields. Simply put, it states that 80% of any observed effect is due to only 20% of the possible causes. When faced with many possible causes of poor performance, constructing a Pareto chart helps us identify which causes are mostly responsible. This in turn allows us to focus improvement efforts on the so-called "vital few" as opposed to the "trivial many." To construct a Pareto chart, the process in question must be observed and a tally made of the frequency with which various possible causes actually result in poor outcome. The chart itself is essentially a vertical bar graph. The various causes are listed across the x-axis of a graph, with bars of equal width placed over each cause, with

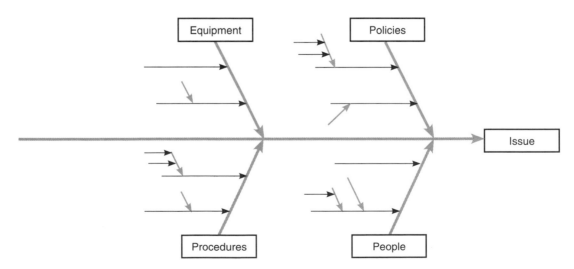

Fig. 5-5. Example of a Fishbone or Ishikawa Diagram.

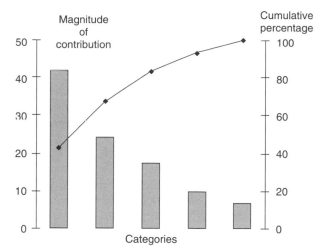

Fig. 5-6. Example of a Pareto Chart.

a height corresponding to the frequency of occurrence. The bars are arranged in descending height order, with the tallest to the left. The left y-axis is the frequency of occurrence, and the right y-axis is labeled with cumulative percentage of occurrences, from 0% to 100%. A curve is then constructed over the bars indicating the cumulative percentage of occurrences with each additional cause, proceeding left to right. A number of very infrequent causes can be pooled together in an "other" category for simplicity. When constructed in this fashion, a Pareto chart often plainly illustrates which two or three causes are responsible for most of the poor outcomes. These causes are where the quality improvement and process redesign efforts should be directed.

The overall purpose of the tools described previously is to allow physicians and administrators to appropriately track the quality of care processes and their outcomes within an obstetric–gynecologic clinical practice setting. Their use will allow detection of deterioration (or improvement) in quality, as well as provide a guide to determining how to correct quality problems.

The following clinical example will illustrate these concepts: Hospital departments of obstetrics and gynecology frequently track postoperative wound infections as a quality indicator. A committee will look at the monthly rate in a table format. Some months the rate is higher, some months lower, but looking at individual months makes it almost impossible to detect trends that may indicate a problem. Plotting the monthly infection rate on a run chart or control chart that is updated at each monthly meeting would allow committee members to quickly determine whether the "infection control" process in the hospital is doing its job. If the run chart or control chart showed evidence of a special cause variation (ie, a single spike beyond the upper control limit or a series of monthly infection rates above the median), then an investigation would be launched to discover the cause. For example, it may turn out that

an autoclave in central supply was malfunctioning, or newly hired personnel in the operating room were not sufficiently trained in sterilization techniques. Correction of this kind of special cause would be seen in the return of the run chart values to normal oscillations around the median. However, when there is no special cause present, the department may decide that its infection rate is too high and needs to be improved. In that case, a cause and effect diagram could be constructed that identified all the components of the process that promote sterility of the operating environment and the reduction of bacterial exposure postoperatively. The wound infection cases would then be analyzed to see which factors are present that might have accounted for those infections. These possible factors would then be graphed in terms of frequency on a Pareto chart, and a decision made to address the two or three most common factors. Perhaps an analysis shows that most of the cases of wound infection did not receive prophylactic antibiotics in the appropriate time frame, and that handwashing by physicians on the postoperative ward was deficient. Protocols would then be developed or strengthened to address these specific issues. If successful, over time these efforts should show a sustained decrease in infection rates on the monthly run charts or control charts as they are reviewed. A point will eventually be reached where the median and control limits will be adjusted downward to reflect the new steady state. The committee could then consider whether to do another round of improvement as part of an ongoing quality measurement cycle.

Quality Measurement Tools

Quality measurement should determine whether the processes of care provided to a single patient or population of patients achieved good outcomes (outcomes measurement) or represented those processes that are thought or known to be associated with achievement of good outcomes (process measurement). Discussed as follows are tools used for quality measurement.

Plan–Do–Study–Act

An important tool for use in quality measurement is the Plan–Do–Study–Act (PDSA) cycle (Fig. 5-7). The PDSA cycle can be used to test changes by planning an intervention, trying the new process, observing the results, and acting on what is learned. It is a scientific method used for action-oriented learning as follows (3):

Plan—Plan the intervention, including a plan for collecting data.

- State the objective of the intervention
- Make predictions about what will happen and why
- Develop a plan to test the change (Who? What? When? Where? What data need to be collected?)

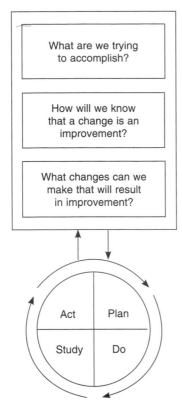

Fig. 5-7. Plan–Do–Study–Act Cycle. (Cambridge, Massachusetts: Institute for Healthcare Improvement; 2009.) (Available on www.IHI.org)

Do—Try out the test on a small scale.

- Carry out the test
- Document problems and unexpected observations
- Begin analysis of the data

Study—Set aside time to analyze the data and study the results.

- Complete the analysis of the data
- Compare the data to predictions
- Summarize and reflect on what was learned

Act—Refine the change, based on what was learned from the test.

- Determine what modifications should be made
- Prepare a plan for the next test

Six Sigma and Lean

Six Sigma is the name given to a management system aimed at reducing variation in manufacturing outputs. Initially developed at Motorola in the 1980s, the name derives from the concept that vigorous process improvement efforts could reduce variability in a manufacturing process such that a full 6 SD of output would still fall within a narrow range of expected performance tolerances. This translates to only three to four defective outputs per million produced, or in the terminology of Six Sigma: three to four defects per million opportunities. This concept and approach was soon adopted by many companies in various industries. It was applied to any process that required improvement, and defects came to represent any outcome that did not meet customer expectations. In health care, one of the few processes that comes close to this "Six Sigma reliability" is mortality from general anesthesia (4).

Six Sigma did not actually introduce any radically new ideas or tools into the field of quality improvement, but, in fact, relies on all the same tools introduced previously. Six Sigma is simply a rigorous application of measurement and data analysis to process evaluation. It focuses on understanding what customer expectations really are, and it directs quality improvement efforts toward what is most important in the eyes of the customer. Lastly, it relies on a commitment to quality improvement from everyone in the organization, particularly top management. To this end, management commits to training individuals whose sole job in the organization becomes devising and implementing process improvement projects. Six Sigma projects are typically divided into five steps as follows:

1. *Define*—Multiple techniques are used to clearly define customers' outcome expectations. Processes to produce these outputs are defined and broken down into component steps.

2. *Measure*—Data is collected around how these process steps contribute to defective outcomes.

3. *Analyze*—Data are analyzed using histograms, run charts, Pareto diagrams, and other tools to determine where the process can best be improved to reduce defective outcomes.

4. *Improve*—Potential solutions are devised, tested, implemented and, most importantly, measured.

5. *Control*—After the desired reduction in defective outcomes is achieved, the effective changes are made permanent and then continually monitored to maintain the improvement over the long term.

Lean, also called "Lean manufacturing" or "Lean production," is another approach to process improvement. It was developed by the Toyota Company and popularized by James Womack in his study of Japanese manufacturing published in 1989 called "Lean Thinking." It focuses on the elimination of waste (called "muda" in Japanese), where waste is defined as anything that does not directly contribute to meeting the customers' requirements. Waste can be in the form of time, energy, defective work, or anything that does not contribute to customer satisfaction. Lean focuses on smooth process flow, reduction of inventories, and just-in-time supply of raw materials to reduce waiting times and wasted effort. This is done while still being flexible to changing customer demands and being open to suggestions for process improvement from anyone in the work force, especially people at the front lines. Lean also makes use of all the quality improvement tools previously discussed. It is sometimes combined with a Six Sigma approach to yield a hybrid approach called "Lean Six Sigma."

Six Sigma is a methodology to improve quality by minimizing variation in a process, and Lean is a methodology to improve quality by reducing waste and reducing the time required to produce results. The two methodologies are not mutually exclusive and are sometimes combined in a single quality improvement project. For example, these concepts have been applied to the development of standardized order sheets for laboratory tests for patients with various conditions presenting to the labor and delivery area. This standardization reduced the omission of necessary tests and the ordering of unnecessary tests, as well as reducing costs. Standardized order sheets also can reduce medication errors, and the application of Lean concepts to a clinical laboratory can reduce reporting time for testing results (5). Many areas of clinical care are amenable to process redesign and outcome improvement through the use of Six Sigma and Lean.

In looking at any of these methods for performance improvement, it should be understood that improvements cannot be made without measurement. Measurements help correct those defects that contribute the most to poor outcomes. Finally, appropriate measures are critical to determine whether a given intervention is having the desired result and improving the process.

Failure Mode and Effects Analysis

Failure Mode and Effects Analysis (FMEA) and Root Cause Analysis (RCA) are tools that may be used in the process of setting up systems or procedures in order to evaluate these systems for possible errors. They may also be used for continued surveillance of ongoing systems and procedures to effect change and corrective actions designed to make them safer.

Failure mode and effects analysis is a tool that is used to analyze proposed systems, production lines, or processes for possible unanticipated faults, defects, and errors. This tool generally is used during the planning or organizing process for these systems or procedures. The potential errors or faults are identified and rated by levels of severity or potential harm that they may cause. This tool also assesses the effect of these errors on the system or procedure that is being considered.

Failure mode and effects analysis was initially used by the military and in aerospace development. It is widely used in manufacturing industries in various phases of production. Medical device and drug delivery systems have added FMEA procedures as a means to understand the potential risks and defects that may not be considered by individual designers. Failure mode and effects analysis is now increasingly finding use in the service industry, and hospitals also have begun to use this technique to prevent the possibility of process errors and mistakes leading to incorrect surgery or medication administration. This use is driven by the Joint Commission.

Failure mode and effects analysis allows a team of persons to review the design or process at key points in its development and make comments and changes to the design of the system or process well in advance of actually experiencing the failure. The U.S. Food and Drug Administration has recognized FMEA as a design verification method for drugs and medical devices.

In an FMEA, failures and errors are prioritized according to how serious their consequences are, how frequently they occur, and how easily they can be detected. An FMEA also documents and updates current knowledge about the process being monitored and is used as a tool for continuous improvement. Failure mode and effects analysis begins during the earliest conceptual stages of design of a process or system and then continues throughout the life of that system. It is used during the design stage with an aim to avoid future potential or actual complications and errors. Later it is used for monitoring and modification before and during ongoing operation of the process.

To begin an FMEA, it is necessary to describe the process, such as implementing a new electronic record for tracking test results (Fig. 5-8). Next, a block diagram of the system needs to be created. This diagram gives an overview of the major components or process steps and how they are related. These are called logical relations around which the FMEA can be developed. The block diagram should always be included with the FMEA. Three process steps are involved in determining a critical index score, which indicates priority areas for correction.

Step 1. Severity

Each effect is given a severity score (S) from 1 to 5. The higher the severity scores, the greater the potential for harm to the customer or patient. These numbers help a designer prioritize the failure modes and their effects. If the severity of an effect has a score of 4 or 5, changes to the design need to be considered by eliminating the failure mode, if possible, or protecting the user from the effect of these failures. A severity score of 4 or 5 generally is reserved for those effects that would cause injury to a user or otherwise result in litigation.

Step 2. Probability

A failure mode is given a probability number from 1 to 5. Actions need to be determined if the occurrence is frequent; for example, a probability score of 3 or more for unsafe or low severity scored errors might require action.

A high severity score, such as 4 or 5, might require action even though it may be relatively infrequent in occurrence with a probability score of 1. Because of the potential for a significant error causing harm even though it occurs infrequently, some corrective action or modification would be appropriate.

Step 3. Detectability

Each combination from the previous two steps that represent potential errors or faults receives a detection number. This number represents the ability of monitoring techniques, tests, and inspections to assess the procedure or system in question to detect any potential error or fault.

After determining the severity, probability, and detectability, the critical index score is calculated by multiplying these three scores: Critical index score = Severity × Probability × Detectability.

Risk priority numbers do not play an important part in the choice of an action against failure modes. Rather, they are threshold values used in the evaluation of these actions in determining priorities for resources and actions to be taken to correct a system or process. This has to be done for the entire process and design. Once this is done, it is easy to determine the areas of greatest concern. The failure modes that have the highest critical index score generally should be given the highest priority for corrective action. This means it is not always the failure modes with the highest severity numbers that should be treated first. There could be less severe failures that occur more often and are less detectable that should be addressed initially.

After these values are allocated, recommended actions with targets, responsibility, and dates of implementation are noted. The FMEA should be updated when any new process or product is introduced that might meet preestablished criteria for conducting the study. Additionally, as an ongoing function, updates should be made whenever changes are made to the operating conditions or

Sample Template											
Problem:							**Date Completed:**				
Team Members:			**Current Status Scores**								
			Severity 1 = no patient harm / 5 = permanent patient harm or death								
			Probability 1 = it is highly unlikely/has never happened before / 5 = it is very likely/it happens quite frequently								
			Detectability 1 = it is highly unlikely / 5 = it is very likely								
			Critical Index (CI) score: Severity × Probability × Detectability								
			Current status scores				Complete for high priority failures				
Process steps	Failure mode	Effect of failure	Severity	Probability	Detectability	CI score	High priority? Y/N	Root causes	Recommended corrective actions	Completion data	Success measures

Fig. 5-8. Diagrammatic representation of an FMEA. (Reprinted from AORN Journal, 78, Spath PL, Using failure mode and effects analysis to improve patient safety, 15–37, July 2003, with permission from Elsevier.)

design of the system or process. Finally, new regulations or customer feedback indicating a problem should trigger a new FMEA.

It is important to note that the success of an FMEA depends on the expertise of the individuals who are setting up the analysis and their familiarity with the systems being evaluated. This is why consideration should be given to having a multidisciplinary team conduct FMEA whenever possible.

The Department of Veterans Affairs National Center for Patient Safety developed a hybrid prospective risk analysis system, Health Care Failure Mode and Effect Analysis, which includes a five-step process that uses an interdisciplinary team to proactively evaluate a health care process. The team uses process flow diagramming, a Hazard Scoring Matrix, and the Health Care Failure Mode and Effect Analysis Decision Tree to identify and assess potential vulnerabilities. Information on this system is publically available through the National Center for Patient Safety (6).

Root Cause Analysis

Root cause analysis is a group of problem-solving methods aimed at identifying the underlying causes of problems or events. The theory of root cause analysis is that problems are best solved by correcting or eliminating root (underlying) causes of the problem and not merely addressing the obvious symptoms. The use of this tool is generally considered in evaluating established systems or procedures as an ongoing modification and correction process.

By directing corrective measures at root causes, one hopes to minimize the likelihood of recurrence. Root cause analysis should be viewed as a process that is similar to that of diagnosing a disease. In looking at the symptom of a disease as the problem, a physician would tend to work backward from "disease state" through the symptoms until the root cause or causes, along with any contributing factors, are determined. Root cause analysis is a tool used to identify process and system failures that result in sentinel events, medical error, or near misses. An RCA should identify the root cause, an identified reason for the presence of a defect or problem, that if eliminated, would prevent recurrence.

There are several general principles that apply to an RCA. The process is a retrospective tool that is applied systemically. It is also an interdisciplinary tool and is performed with the ultimate goal of concentrating on the systems and processes rather than the performance of individuals. It is a learning tool that is used to promote teamwork, facilitate open communication, prevent similar errors in the future, and enhance patient safety and quality of care. Relevant data and literature must be used in drawing conclusions that are evidence based. There is frequently more than one root cause for any given problem. This tool looks into determining human factors as

well as related processes and systems. There is recognition that complete prevention of recurrence of an error by a single intervention is not always possible, and as a result, an RCA often is considered to be an iterative process and viewed as a tool of continuous improvement. There are generally seven steps in performing an RCA.

Step 1. Forming an RCA Team

There are different approaches to establishing this team and each institution must decide which approach works best for its organization. One method is for the organization to have a standing RCA team that is available to respond to any type of sentinel event and, if appropriate, other medical errors and near misses. This type of approach allows for an efficient and consistent approach to performing an RCA by a team that is experienced in the process. The negative aspect of this approach, however, is that the people on the front line are usually in the best position to identify issues and solutions, and an established RCA team that does not include these individuals might not have as much insight in investigating an error. If the institution does not include all individuals involved in, and leading up to, the incident, it is important to communicate results and changes to them when the RCA is completed.

Another method is to establish an ad hoc team in response to a sentinel event. This allows the use of front-line individuals who may have a better insight into the process being analyzed. Some potential participants may include a physician, nurse, pharmacist, social worker, administrator, risk manager, quality improvement analyst, patient (member of community), and information systems representative. The ultimate composition of the team will depend on the event being analyzed. However, a more common method is a combination of the previously discussed methods.

An additional decision that needs to be made is whether individuals involved in the event should participate on the RCA team. On the one hand, benefits for their inclusion are that caregivers are allowed to heal by their ability to look at the problem from a systems perspective rather than assigning individual blame. They also have first-hand understanding of how to prevent recurrence. On the other hand, their inclusion may inhibit the free flow of information by making the caregiver feel uncomfortable talking about the event because of stress or trauma. Regardless of the decision about caregiver participation on the RCA team, all efforts should be made to value each member's opinions equally, putting aside rank. This atmosphere must be reinforced by the team leader.

Using a facilitator as part of the team is also helpful since the facilitator would assist in setting and enforcing ground rules and make the environment safe for disclosure because RCAs can be emotional and threatening events. The facilitator would also be able to keep the group focused on digging for the root cause or causes and assuring that the action plan addresses the identified root cause or causes. The use of a facilitator also provides a leader for the RCA team.

Step 2. Identify the Problem

An RCA team establishes the scope of the analysis, defines the problem that is to be investigated, and keeps the analysis focused and simple. Putting this in writing may be helpful. Often, a sentinel event or a near miss may present with several possible issues that may be investigated, but it helps to focus the process on a specific problem.

Step 3. Gather Information and Evidence

Information collection generally is done by interviewing all who are involved in the event as part of the RCA process. All collected information should be documented thoroughly. The collected information should be presented to the RCA team and follow up if needed for additional information or clarification after going over the initial findings with the RCA team. As the interviews and information gathering proceeds, additional side observations may become apparent. These may not have an effect on the current investigation, but they may be important in other aspects of patient care and could be used to correct or improve other processes. During this step, ideas that are not relevant to the current issue should be placed in a "parking lot," a temporary holding area for ideas or suggestions that are not directly on-topic with the issue facing the group. These issues may then be addressed at a later time.

There are two types of flow charts that may be utilized to track an event and record the information gathered. One method of representing a process leading to an adverse event or possible sentinel event is the "fishbone diagram." In this representation (Fig. 5-9), the events leading up to the eventual outcome are represented by a linear arrow. The spines of the fishbone represent the various system components that are part of the process and affect the event. The underlying drivers are the built-in system regulations or actions that tend to drive the system to the eventual outcome. In the case of an adverse or sentinel event, these represent poorly designed processes that may have likely led to a poor outcome. The countermeasures represent built-in or ad hoc processes that tend to prevent the progression of actions that might ultimately lead to a poor outcome.

Another method of evaluating an adverse event is to use a block style template. By working backwards, the steps that are part of a sequence of events that ultimately lead to the error or sentinel event can be identified. This technique has been criticized as being too basic to analyze root causes because the questions asked are limited by the knowledge of the persons asking the questions. Also, the results are not repeatable—different people using the "'Five Whys" model come up with different causes for the same problem. By repeatedly asking the question "Why?" five times, the layers of symptoms are gradually peeled away, which can then lead to the root cause of the problem. Additionally, there may be multiple causes for a sentinel event which are not represented in this model.

Step 4. Determining Root Causes or Relevant Events

After the data are gathered and entered into a diagrammatic representation, it is important to determine the relevance of the information gathered (Fig. 5-10). Does the information gathered describe the process in question, and is it relevant to the problem being investigated? The question that is posed for each step should be, "Did this action contribute to the eventual error?" Consider how possible root causes are related and how likely correction or elimination of the possible root causes will prevent recurrence.

The first four steps of this process involve determining the root cause of a particular problem, such as implementing a new electronic system for test results. The root

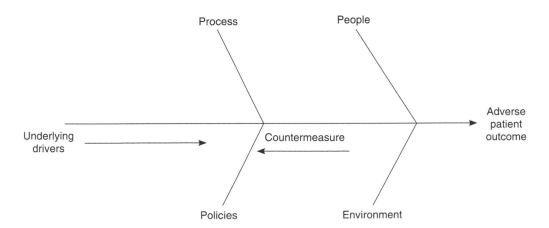

Fig. 5-9. Fishbone Diagram of an Event.

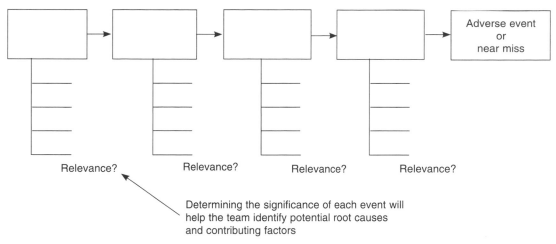

Relevance? Relevance? Relevance? Relevance?

Determining the significance of each event will
help the team identify potential root causes
and contributing factors

Fig. 5-10. Sample Template for Developing a Root Cause Analysis.

causes may appear to be self-evident, but by following a process of continuing to ask the "Five Why's" after each apparent cause, groups generally find root causes that, when changed, truly reduce the risk of a repeat of the event. For example, in analyzing a case of a prolapsed umbilical cord after spontaneous rupture of membranes in which the decision to incision time was 40 minutes, the group might stop at "anesthesiologist was not in house." By continuing to ask "Why?", the group might find that this treatment delay was related to any number of causes: staffing levels, orientation and training of staff, staff supervision, communication among staff members, and availability of information. The last three steps demonstrate the actions taken as a result of determining the root cause of a problem and implementing changes in the process being evaluated.

Step 5. Explore Risk Reduction and Quality Improvement Strategies

When the search for the root causes of an error is completed, the process of analyzing possible solutions begins. This step is essentially a brainstorming session that explores options to correct problems that have been uncovered. For each problem discovered, a possible solution is presented.

Step 6. Implement a Redesign Template

After the root causes of an adverse event have been identified and potential alternate solutions and strategies have been developed, their implementation can be explored. Some solutions may be easier to implement than others if fewer resources are required. The group must set priorities so that changes that may have a large effect on eliminating errors are done first, while less effective plans are assigned a lower priority. Additionally, the redesign needs to determine where altering current processes will expose the process being analyzed to other unanticipated errors.

Step 7. Monitor and Evaluate New Systems

Once the new processes have been implemented, continued surveillance must be carried out to determine whether the new process has eliminated the identified errors and has not exposed the system to alternate adverse events. The group must decide as part of the RCA process who will be accountable for this activity. Measures should be developed that will allow an ongoing evaluation of the effectiveness of the new process. Outcomes of ongoing measurement should be reported so that the RCA can be used as a learning opportunity for the entire organization.

Regulatory Requirements for Root Cause Analysis

Performing an RCA is often triggered as a requirement of the Joint Commission. In addition to the Joint Commission, there may be other state and local regulatory agencies that could require an RCA in response to a medical error or some other poor outcome. In some cases, a medical liability carrier might require an RCA as a result of a poor patient outcome that could potentially increase a liability exposure for the carrier and its clients.

Listed are some examples of sentinel events that are reviewable under the Joint Commission's Sentinel Event Policy:

- Any patient death associated with a medication error
- Any intrapartum (birth-related) maternal death
- Any perinatal death unrelated to a congenital condition in an infant having a birth weight greater than 2,500 grams
- A patient abduction from the hospital where he or she receives care, treatment, or services
- Hemolytic transfusion reaction involving major blood group incompatibilities

- A foreign body, such as a sponge or forceps, that was left in a patient after surgery

The Joint Commission has a list of specific sentinel events that require that an RCA be performed. The Joint Commission requires that specific sentinel events that trigger an RCA include an evaluation of very specific processes as part of the RCA (7). The hospital should incorporate the RCA and its resultant monitoring into the ongoing quality improvement process.

References

1. Carey RG, Lloyd RC. Measuring quality improvement in healthcare: a guide to statistical process control applications. Milwaukee (WI): American Society for Quality; 2001.
2. Ransom SB, Joshi M, Nash DB. The healthcare quality book: vision, strategy, and tools. Health Administration Press: Chicago (IL); 2005.
3. Langley GJ, Moen RD, Nolan KM, Nolan TW, Norman CL, Provost LP. The improvement guide: a practical approach to enhancing organizational performance. 2nd ed. Jossey-Bass: San Francisco (CA); 2009.
4. Pande PS, Neuman RP, Cavanagh RR. The Six Sigma way: how GE, Motorola, and other top companies are honing their performance. New York (NY): McGraw-Hill; 2000.
5. Chassin R. The Six Sigma initiative at Mount Sinai Medical Center. Mt Sinai J Med 2008;75:45–52.
6. Department of Veterans Affairs, National Center for Patient Safety. Healthcare failure mode and effect analysis (HFMEA™). Ann Arbor (MI): NCPS; 2009. Available at: http://www.patientsafety.gov/SafetyTopics.html#HFMEA. Retrieved June 29, 2009.
7. The Joint Commission. Sentinel event policy and procedures. Oakbrook Terrace (IL): JC; 2007. Available at: http://www.jointcommission.org/NR/rdonlyres/F84F9DC6-A5DA-490F-A91F-A9FCE26347C4/0/SE_chapter_july07.pdf. Retrieved June 18, 2009.

Additional Resources

Department of Veterans Affairs, National Center for Patient Safety. Root cause analysis. Ann Arbor (MI): NCPS; 2009. Available at: http://www.va.gov/ncps/vision.html#RCA. Retrieved June 18, 2009.

Joint Commission Resources. Engaging physicians in patient safety: a handbook for leaders. Oakbrook Terrace (IL): Joint Commission on Accreditation of Healthcare Organizations; 2006.

Joint Commission Resources. Root cause analysis in health care: tools and techniques. 4th ed. Oakbrook Terrace (IL): Joint Commission on Accreditation of Healthcare Organizations; 2009.

Lighter DE, Fair DC. Quality management in health care: principles and methods. Subury (MA): Jones and Bartlett; 2004.

Quality Associates International. FMEA (Failure Mode and Effects Analysis). Available at: http://www.quality-one.com/services/fmea.php.

APPENDIX A

Glossary

Action plan—The product of the root cause analysis that identifies the strategies that an organization intends to implement to reduce the risk of similar events occurring in the future. The plan should address responsibility for implementation, oversight, pilot testing as appropriate, timelines, and strategies for measuring the effectiveness of the actions.

Adverse drug event (ADE)—An adverse event involving medication use.

Examples:

- anaphylaxis to penicillin
- major hemorrhage from heparin
- aminoglycoside-induced renal failure
- agranulocytosis from chloramphenicol

As with the more general term adverse event, there is no necessary relation to error or poor quality of care. In other words, ADEs include expected adverse drug reactions (or side effects), as well as events due to error.

Thus, a serious allergic reaction to penicillin in a patient with no prior such history is an ADE, but so is the same reaction in a patient who does have a known allergy history but receives penicillin due to a prescribing oversight. To avoid having to use medication error as an outcome, some studies refer instead to potential ADEs. For instance, if a clinician ordered penicillin for a patient with a documented serious penicillin allergy, many would characterize the order as a potential ADE, on the grounds that administration of the drug would carry a substantial risk of harm to the patient.

Ignoring the distinction between expected medication side effects and ADEs due to errors may seem misleading, but a similar distinction can be achieved with the concept of preventability. All ADEs due to error are preventable, but other ADEs not warranting the label error also may be preventable.

Benchmark—1. A point of reference or standard by which something can be measured, compared, or judged, as in benchmarks of performance. 2. A standard unit for the basis of comparison, that is, a universal unit that is identified with sufficient detail so that other similar classifications can be compared as being above, below, or comparable to the benchmark.

Briefings and debriefings—Similar to a preflight checklist used in aviation, during a brief, the team leader should cover the items on the checklist. Briefings provide the ideal forum for building a team dynamic that allows everyone to work together when carrying out routine tasks and when tackling unexpected problems. The following information should be discussed in a brief: 1) team membership and roles; 2) clinical status of the team's patients; 3) team goals, pitfalls, and barriers; and 4) issues affecting team operations. Debriefings occur after the patient encounter and include: 1) an accurate recounting and documentation of key events; 2) an analysis of why the event occurred, what worked, and what did not work; 3) a discussion of lessons learned and how they will alter the plan next time; and 4) establishment of a method to formally change the existing plan to incorporate lessons learned (1).

Clinical pathway—A treatment regimen, agreed on by consensus, that includes all the elements of care, regardless of the effect on patient outcomes. It is a broader look at care and may include tests and X-rays that do not affect patient recovery.

Computerized Physician Order Entry or Computerized Provider Order Entry (CPOE)—Refers to a computer-based system of ordering medications and often other tests. Physicians (or other providers) directly enter orders into a computer system that can have varying levels of sophistication. Basic CPOE ensures standardized, legible, complete orders, and thus, reduces errors due to poor handwriting and ambiguous abbreviations. Almost all CPOE systems offer some additional capabilities, which fall under the general rubric of Clinical Decision Support System (CDSS). Typical CDSS features involve suggested default values for drug doses, routes of administration, or frequency. More sophisticated CDSSs can perform drug allergy checks (eg, the user orders ceftriaxone and a warning flashes that the patient has a documented penicillin allergy), drug–laboratory value checks (eg, initiating an order for gentamicin prompts the system to alert the health care provider to the patient's last creatinine measurement), or drug–drug interaction checks. At the highest level of sophistication, CDSS prevents not only errors of commission (eg, ordering a drug in excessive doses or in the setting of a serious allergy), but also of omission. (For example, an alert may appear such as, "You have ordered heparin; would you like to order a PTT in 6 hours?" or, an even more sophisticated alert: "The admitting diagnosis is hip fracture; would you like to order heparin DVT prophylaxis?")

Construct validity—Refers to the ability of the instrument to measure the "hypothetical construct" at the heart of what is being measured. Where a gold standard does not exist (as is the case for measuring humanistic qualities such as compassion, integrity, responsibility, and respect), construct validity is determined by designing experiments that explore the ability of the instrument to "measure" the construct in question. This is often done by applying the scale to different populations that are known to have differing amounts of the property to be assessed. By conducting a series of converging studies, the construct validity of the new instrument can be determined.

Continuous quality improvement—A set of techniques for continuous study and improvement of the processes of delivering health care services and products to meet the needs and expectations of the customers of those services and products. It has three basic elements: 1) customer knowledge, 2) a focus on processes of health care delivery, and 3) statistical approaches that aim to reduce variations in those processes.

Credentialing—The process of obtaining, verifying, and assessing the qualifications of a health care practitioner to provide patient care services in or for a health care organization. The determination is based on an evaluation of the individual's current license, education, training, experience, competence, and professional judgment. The process is the basis for making appointments to the professional staff of a health care organization. The process also provides information for granting clinical privileges to licensed independent practitioners.

Disruptive behavior—An aberrant style of personal interaction with physicians, hospital personnel, patients, family members, or others that potentially interferes with patient care.

Due process—The right of fundamental fairness in proceedings. Procedural due process requires that notice and right to a fair hearing be afforded before an action is taken that might deprive an individual of his or her property or liberty.

Error—An act of commission (doing something wrong) or omission (failing to do the right thing) that leads to an undesirable outcome or significant potential for such an outcome. For instance, ordering a medication for a patient with a documented allergy to that medication would be an act of commission. Failing to prescribe a proven medication with major benefits for an eligible patient (eg, low-dose unfractionated heparin as venous thromboembolism prophylaxis for a patient after hip replacement surgery) would represent an error of omission.

Errors of omission are more difficult to recognize than errors of commission but likely represent a larger problem. In other words, there are likely many more instances in which the provision of additional diagnostic, therapeutic, or preventive modalities would have improved care than there are instances in which the care provided quite literally should not have been provided. In many ways, this point echoes the generally agreed-upon view in health care quality literature that underuse far exceeds overuse, even though the latter historically received greater attention.

In addition to commission versus omission, three other dichotomies commonly appear in literature on errors: active failures versus latent conditions, errors at the "sharp end" versus errors at the "blunt end," and slips versus mistakes.

Face validity—Indicates whether an instrument seems to either the users or designers to be assessing the correct qualities. It is essentially a subjective judgment.

Facilitator—In quality improvement (QI), a person who has developed special expertise in the QI process. He or she does not belong to a QI team but helps it achieve results by helping to focus its efforts, teaching QI methods, consulting with the team leader, and helping connect the work to the knowledge necessary for improvement.

The Five Rights—The "Five Rights"—administering the Right Medication, in the Right Dose, at the Right Time, by the Right Route, to the Right Patient—are the cornerstone of traditional nursing teaching about safe medication practice.

Forcing function—An aspect of a design that prevents a target action from being performed or allows its performance only if another specific action is performed first. For example, automobiles are now designed so that the driver cannot shift into reverse without first putting her foot on the brake pedal. Forcing functions need not involve device design. For instance, one of the first forcing functions identified in health care is the removal of concentrated potassium from general hospital wards. This action is intended to prevent the inadvertent preparation of intravenous solutions with concentrated potassium, an error that has produced small but consistent numbers of deaths for many years.

Health literacy—Individuals' ability to find, process, and comprehend the basic health information necessary to act on medical instructions and make decisions about their health (2).

High Reliability Organizations (HROs)—High reliability organizations refer to organizations or systems that operate in hazardous conditions but have fewer adverse events (3, 4). Commonly discussed examples include air traffic control systems, nuclear power plants, and naval aircraft carriers (5, 6). It is worth noting that, in patient safety literature, HROs are considered to operate with nearly failure-free performance records, not simply better than average ones. This shift in meaning is somewhat understandable given that the failure rates in these other industries are so much lower than rates of errors and adverse events in health care. This comparison glosses over the difference in significance of a failure in the nuclear power industry compared with one in health care. The point remains, however, that some organizations achieve consistently safe and effective performance records despite unpredictable operating environments or intrinsically hazardous endeavors. Detailed case studies of specific HROs have identified some common features, which have been offered as models for other organizations to achieve substantial improvements in their safety records. These features include:

- Preoccupation with failure—The acknowledgment of the high-risk, error-prone nature of an organization's activities and the determination to achieve consistently safe operations.

- Commitment to resilience—The development of capacities to detect unexpected threats and contain them before they cause harm, or bounce back when they do.

- Sensitivity to operations—An attentiveness to the issues facing workers at the front line. This feature comes into play when conducting analyses of specific events (eg, frontline workers play a crucial role in root cause analyses by bringing up unrecognized latent threats in current operating procedures), but also in connection with organizational decision making, which is somewhat decentralized. Management units at the front line are given some autonomy in identifying and responding to threats, rather than adopting a rigid top-down approach.

- A culture of safety in which individuals feel comfortable drawing attention to potential hazards or actual failures without fear of censure from management.

Indicator—1. A measure used to determine, over time, performance of functions, processes, and outcomes. 2. A statistical value that provides an indication of the condition or direction, over time, of performance of a defined process or achievement of a defined outcome.

Informed consent—The process of providing information to patients about the risks and benefits of treatment, as well as alternatives to treatment, before performing any procedure or initiating any treatment.

Informed decision making—An individual's overall process of gathering relevant information from both her clinician and from other clinical and nonclinical sources, with or without independent clarification of values. (*see also* Shared decision making)

Just culture—The phrase "just culture" was popularized in the patient safety lexicon by a report that outlined principles for achieving a culture in which frontline personnel feel comfortable disclosing errors—including their own—while maintaining professional accountability (7). The examples in the report relate to transfusion safety, but the principles clearly generalize across domains within health care organizations.

Traditionally, health care's culture has held individuals accountable for all errors or mishaps that befall patients under their care. By contrast, a just culture recognizes that individual practitioners should not be held accountable for system failings over which they have no control. A just culture also recognizes many individual or active errors represent predictable interactions between human operators and the systems in which they work. However, in contrast to a culture that touts "no blame" as its governing principle, a just culture does not tolerate conscious disregard of clear risks to patients or gross misconduct (eg, falsifying a record or performing professional duties while intoxicated).

In summary, a just culture recognizes that competent professionals make mistakes and acknowledges that even competent professionals will develop unhealthy norms (such as shortcuts or routine rule violations), but has zero tolerance for reckless behavior.

Near miss—An event or situation that did not produce patient injury, but only because of chance; also referred to as a "close call." This good fortune might reflect robustness of the patient (eg, a patient with penicillin allergy receives penicillin, but has no reaction) or a fortuitous, timely intervention (eg, a nurse happens to realize that a physician wrote an order in the wrong chart).

Normalization of deviance—Normalization of deviance was coined by Diane Vaughan in her book, *The Challenger Launch Decision: Risky Technology, Culture, and Deviance at NASA* in which she analyzes the interactions between various cultural forces within NASA that contributed to the Challenger space shuttle disaster (8). Vaughn used this expression to describe the gradual shift in what is regarded as normal after repeated exposures to "deviant behavior" (behavior straying from correct [or safe] operating procedure). Corners get cut, safety checks bypassed, and alarms ignored or turned off, and these behaviors become *normal*—not just common, but stripped of their significance as warnings of impending danger. In their discussion of a catastrophic error in health care, Mark Chassin and Elise Becher used the phrase "a culture of low expectations"(9). When a system routinely produces errors (eg, paperwork in the wrong chart, major miscommunications between different members of a given health care team, patients are not informed about important aspects of their care), health care providers in the system become inured to malfunction. In such a system, what should be regarded as a major warning of impending danger is ignored as a normal operating procedure.

Outcome—Denotes the effects of care on the health status of patients and populations. Improvements in the patient's knowledge and salutary changes in the patient's behavior are included under a broad definition of health status, and so is the degree of the patient's satisfaction with care.

Outliers—1. Any measurement that is beyond a predetermined threshold of appropriate care. 2. Health care providers with performance or outcome rates that are outside the range of expected rates after adjustment for patient or other characteristics.

Patient safety—Freedom from accidental or preventable injuries produced by medical care.

Performance measures—Methods or instruments to estimate or monitor the extent to which the actions of a health care practitioner or provider conform to the clinical practice guideline.

Physician impairment—The inability of a physician to practice medicine with reasonable skill and with safety to patients due to a disability, such as alcohol or drug abuse, mental illness, handicap, or senility.

Plan–Do–Study–Act (PDSA) cycle—A four-part method for discovering and correcting assignable causes to improve the quality of processes. Modification of the Plan–Do–Check–Act cycle.

Practice guidelines—Systematically developed statements to assist practitioner and patient decisions about appropriate health care for specific clinical circumstances.

Preceptorship—An educational program designed to give the professionally trained students experience outside the academic environment working in the specialty area of their choice with a physician or other advisory supervisors.

Privileging—The process whereby a specific scope and content of patient care services (that is, clinical privileges) are authorized for a health care practitioner by a health care organization based on evaluation of the individual's credentials and performance.

Proctoring—Observation and evaluation of a practitioner for appointment or clinical privileges.

Process—Denotes what is actually done in giving and receiving care. It includes the patient's activities in seeking care and carrying it out as well as the practitioner's activities in making a diagnosis and recommending or implementing treatment.

Quality improvement—The attainment, or process of attaining, a new level of performance or quality that is superior to any previous level of quality.

Read-backs—When information is conveyed verbally, miscommunication may occur in a variety of ways, especially when transmission may not occur clearly (eg, by telephone or radio, or if communication occurs under stress). For names and numbers, the problem often is confusing the sound of one letter or number with another. To address this possibility, the military, civil aviation, and many high-risk industries use protocols for mandatory "read-backs," in which the listener repeats the key information, so that the transmitter can confirm that it is correct.

Because mistaken substitution or reversal of alphanumeric information is such a potential hazard, read-back protocols typically include the use of phonetic alphabets, such as the NATO system ("*Alpha-Bravo-Charlie-Delta-Echo...X-ray-Yankee-Zulu*") now familiar to many people. In health care, traditionally, read-back has been mandatory only in the context of checking to ensure accurate identification of recipients of blood transfusions. However, there are many other circumstances in which health care teams could benefit from following such protocols, for example, when communicating key lab results or patient orders over the phone, and even when exchanging information in person (eg, "sign outs" and other such handoffs).

Recredentialing—The process of determining and certifying the competence of a physician or other professional at some time after the initial determination of his or her qualification for licensure or hospital privileges. Recredentialing is required at periodic intervals (such as every 2 years) in most hospitals and other types of health care organizations. Recredentialing focuses on physicians' actual performance, rather than on physicians' capacity to perform well, as reflected, for example, in passing a written examination.

Safety culture—Safety culture and culture of safety are frequently encountered terms referring to a commitment to safety that permeates all levels of an organization, from frontline personnel to executive management. More specifically, safety culture calls up a number of features identified in studies of high reliability organizations, organizations outside of health care with exemplary performance with respect to safety (6, 10). These features include (11):

- acknowledgment of the high-risk, error-prone nature of an organization's activities
- a blame-free environment where individuals are able to report errors or close calls without fear of reprimand or punishment
- an expectation of collaboration across ranks to seek solutions to vulnerabilities
- a willingness on the part of the organization to direct resources for addressing safety concerns

The Veterans Affairs system has explicitly focused on achieving a culture of safety, in addition to its focus on a number of specific patient safety initiatives (12). The effect of such efforts are difficult to assess, but some tools for quantifying the degree to which organizations differ with respect to "safety culture" have begun to emerge (13).

Sentinel event—An adverse event in which death or serious harm to a patient has occurred; usually used to refer to events that are not at all expected or acceptable (eg, an operation on the wrong patient or body part). The choice of the word "sentinel" reflects the egregiousness of the injury (eg, amputation of the wrong leg) and the likelihood that investigation of such events will reveal serious problems in current policies or procedures.

Shared decision making—Goes beyond informed decision making by emphasizing that the decision process is joint and shared between the patient and health care provider. (*See also* Informed decision making)

Sharp end—The "sharp end" refers to the personnel or parts of the health care system in direct contact with patients. Personnel operating at the sharp end may literally be holding a scalpel (eg, an orthopedist who operates on the wrong leg) or figuratively be administering any kind of therapy (eg, a nurse programming an intravenous pump) or performing any aspect of care.

To complete the metaphor, the "blunt end" refers to the many layers of the health care system that affect the scalpels, pills, and medical devices, or the personnel wielding, administering, and operating them.

Thus, an error in programming an intravenous pump would represent a problem at the sharp end, while the institution's decision to use multiple types of infusion pumps (making programming errors more likely) would represent a problem at the blunt end.

Structure-Process-Outcome Triad—Quality has been defined as the "degree to which health services for individuals and populations increase the likelihood of desired health outcomes and are consistent with current professional knowledge" (14). This definition, like most others, emphasizes favorable patient outcomes as the gold standard for assessing quality. In practice, however, one would like to detect quality problems without waiting for poor outcomes to develop in such sufficient numbers that deviations from expected rates of morbidity and mortality can be detected. Avedis Donabedian first proposed that quality could be measured using aspects of care with proven relationships to desirable patient outcomes (15, 16). For instance, if proven diagnostic and therapeutic strategies are monitored, quality problems can be detected long before demonstrable poor outcomes occur.

Aspects of care with proven connections to patient outcomes fall into two general categories: process and structure. Processes encompass all that is done to patients in terms of diagnosis, treatment, monitoring, and counseling. Cardiovascular care provides classic examples of the use of process measures to assess quality. Given the known benefits of aspirin and beta-blockers for patients with myocardial infarction, the quality of care for patients with myocardial infarction can be measured in terms of the rates at which eligible patients receive these proven therapies. The percentage of eligible women who undergo mammography at appropriate intervals would provide a process-based measure for quality of preventive care for women.

Structure refers to the setting in which care occurs and the capacity of that setting to produce quality. Traditional examples of structural measures related to quality include credentials, patient volume, and academic affiliation. More recent structural measures include the adoption of organizational models for inpatient care (eg, closed intensive care units and dedicated stroke units) and possibly the presence of sophisticated clinical information systems. Cardiovascular care provides another classic example of structural measures of quality. Numerous studies have shown that institutions that perform more cardiac surgeries and invasive cardiology procedures achieve better outcomes than institutions that see fewer patients. Given these data, patient volume represents a structural measure of quality of care for patients undergoing cardiac procedures.

Swiss cheese model—James Reason developed the "Swiss cheese model" (Fig. 1-2) to illustrate how analyses of major accidents and catastrophic systems failures tend to reveal multiple, smaller failures leading up to the actual hazard. In the model, each slice of cheese represents a safety barrier or precaution relevant to a particular hazard. For example, if the hazard was wrong-site surgery, slices of the cheese might include conventions for identifying the side on radiology tests, a protocol for signing the correct site when the surgeon and patient first meet, and a second protocol for reviewing the medical record and checking the previously marked site in the operating room. Many more layers exist. The point is that no single barrier is foolproof. They each have "holes"; hence, the Swiss cheese. For some serious events (eg, operating on the wrong site or wrong person), even though the holes will align infrequently, even rare cases of harm (errors making it "through the cheese") will be unacceptable.

TeamSTEPPS (Strategies and Tools to Enhance Performance and Patient Safety)—An evidence-based teamwork system aimed at optimizing patient outcomes by improving communication and other teamwork skills among health care professionals. TeamSTEPPS includes a comprehensive suite of ready-to-use materials and training curricula necessary to successfully integrate teamwork principles into all areas of the health care system. TeamSTEPPS was developed by the Department of Defense Patient Safety Program, in collaboration with the Agency for Healthcare Research and Quality (1).

Threshold—The level or point at which a stimulus is strong enough to signal the need for response. For example, threshold for pain or threshold for review of an occurrence measured by a clinical indicator.

"Time-outs"—Refer to planned periods of quiet and interdisciplinary discussion focused on ensuring that key procedural details have been addressed. For instance, protocols for ensuring correct site surgery often recommend a "time-out" to confirm the identification of the patient, the surgical procedure, the surgical site, and other key aspects, often stating them aloud for double-checking by other team members. In addition to avoiding major misidentification errors involving the patient or surgical site, such a time-out ensures that all team members share the same "game plan." Taking the time to focus on listening and communicating the plans as a team can rectify miscommunications and misunderstandings before a procedure gets underway.

Two-challenge rule—The two-challenge rule was developed by human factors experts to help airline captains prevent disasters caused when otherwise excellent decision makers experience momentary lapses in judgment. In the clinical environment, team members should challenge colleagues if requesting clarification and confirmation does not alleviate concern regarding potential harm to a patient. If after two attempts the concern is still disregarded, but the member believes patient or staff safety is or may be severely compromised, the two-challenge rule mandates taking a stronger course of action or using a supervisor or chain of command. This overcomes the natural tendency to believe the medical team leader must always know what should be done, even when the actions taken depart from established guidelines. When invoking this rule and moving up the chain, it is essential to communicate to the entire medical team that additional input has been solicited.

Workaround—From the perspective of frontline personnel trying to accomplish their work, the design of equipment or the policies governing work tasks can seem counterproductive. When frontline personnel adopt consistent patterns of work or ways of bypassing safety features of medical equipment, these patterns and actions are referred to as "workarounds." Although workarounds "fix the problem," the system remains unaltered and thus continues to present potential safety hazards for future patients.

Resources

1. Agency for Healthcare Research and Quality. TeamSTEPPS curriculum tools and materials. Available at: http://team-stepps.ahrq.gov/abouttoolsmaterials.htm. Retrieved June 29, 2009.

2. Health literacy: report of the Council on Scientific Affairs. Ad Hoc Committee on Health Literacy for the Council on Scientific Affairs, American Medical Association. JAMA 1999;281:552-7.

3. Weick KE, Sutcliffe KM. Managing the unexpected: resilient performance in an age of uncertainty. 2nd ed. San Francisco (CA): Jossey-Bass; 2007.

4. Reason J. Human error: models and management. BMJ 2000;320:768-70.

5. LaPorte TR. The United States air traffic system: increasing reliability in the midst of rapid growth. In: Mayntz R, Hughes TP, editors. The development of large technical systems. Boulder (CO): Westview Press; 1988. p. 215-44.

6. Roberts KH. Managing high reliability organizations. Calif Manage Rev 1990;32:101-14.

7. Marx D. Patient safety and the "just culture": a primer for health care executives. New York (NY): Trustees of Columbia University in the City of New York; 2001. Available at: http://www.mers-tm.org/support/Marx_Primer.pdf. Retrieved June 29, 2009.

8. Vaughan D. The Challenger launch decision: risky technology, culture, and deviance at NASA. Chicago (IL): University of Chicago Press; 1996.

9. Chassin MR, Becher EC. The wrong patient. Ann Intern Med 2002;136:826-33.

10. Weick KE. Organizational culture as a source of high reliability. Calif Manage Rev 1987;29:112-27.

11. Pizzi LT, Goldfarb NI, Nash DB. Promoting a culture of safety. In: Agency for Healthcare Research and Quality. Making health care safer: a critical analysis of patient safety practices. Evidence Report/Technology Assessment, No. 43. Rockville (MD): AHRQ; 2001. p. 447-57. http://www.ahrq.gov/clinic/ptsafety/pdf/chap40.pdf. Retrieved June 29, 2009.

12. Weeks WB, Bagian JP. Developing a culture of safety in the Veterans Health Administration. Eff Clin Pract 2000; 3:270-6.

13. Singer SJ, Gaba DM, Geppert JJ, Sinaiko AD, Howard SK, Park KC. The culture of safety: results of an organization-wide survey in 15 California hospitals. Qual Saf Health Care 2003;12:112-8.

14. Institute of Medicine (US). Medicare: a strategy for quality assurance. Washington, DC: National Academy Press; 1990.

15. Donabedian A. Evaluating the quality of medical care. Milbank Mem Fund Q 1966;44 suppl:166-206.

16. Donabedian A. Explorations in quality assessment and monitoring. Volume I: the definition of quality and approaches to its assessment. Ann Arbor (MI): Health Administration Press; 1980.

APPENDIX B

Voluntary Review of Quality Care Program Overview

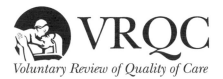

Voluntary Review of Quality of Care

One of the American Congress of Obstetricians and Gynecologists' most successful programs to date is the Voluntary Review of Quality Care (VRQC) Program, established in 1986. The mission of the VRQC Program is to provide peer review consultations to departments of obstetrics and gynecology, assess the quality of care provided, and suggest possible alternative actions for improvement. The program offers comprehensive, department-wide reviews that focus on all practitioners with obstetric–gynecologic privileges.

This is accomplished by way of a site visit conducted by three board-certified, practicing obstetrician–gynecologists and a nurse with experience in obstetrics and gynecology, utilizing various quality assessment techniques, including an evaluation based on the American College of Obstetricians and Gynecologists' guidelines. Reviewers are selected from the VRQC Reviewer Panel, composed of Fellows of the American College of Obstetricians and Gynecologists experienced in peer review and quality assessment techniques; board-certified physicians in other specialties (ie, anesthesiologists and family physicians); certified nurse–midwives; and nurses specializing in obstetrics, customized to meet the needs of the hospital. The hospital is given the opportu-

nity, prior to the site visit, to review credentials of the reviewers chosen.

Based on findings revealed from hospital data, medical record review, and interviews of key hospital staff, the American Congress of Obstetricians and Gynecologists provides a confidential, comprehensive final report for the hospital containing specific recommendations. These reports are valuable tools in promoting constructive changes and helping to identify potential areas for improvement of quality of care provided. Typically, the report contains recommendations on how to improve the system, adopt new programs, and address the hospital's particular concerns.

Programs like the VRQC serve as the foundation to our efforts to ensure quality care. The VRQC Steering Committee updates the data collection forms used for the chart reviews on a continuous basis to keep up-to-date with the most current guidelines on practice management and documentation. These data collection forms, along with instructions on how to use them for chart review, can be accessed through the VRQC web site at: http://www.acog.org/goto/vrqc.

If you would like to learn more about the program, contact the VRQC Manager at vrqc@acog.org or call (800) 266-8043.

APPENDIX C

Measurement Resources

For the most recent measure specifications, standards, or benchmarks, please refer to the following organizations:

Accreditation Association for Ambulatory Health Care
Ambulatory standards and resources for accreditation
5250 Old Orchard Road, Suite 200
Skokie, IL 60077
(847) 853-6060
http://www.aaahc.org

National Quality Measures Clearinghouse™ (NQMC)
Agency for Healthcare Research and Quality
Public repository of evidence-based quality measures and measure sets
Office of Communications and Knowledge Transfer
540 Gaither Road, Suite 2000
Rockville, MD 20850
(301) 427-1364
http://www.qualitymeasures.ahrq.gov

Physician Consortium for Performance Improvement
American Medical Association
Collection of physician-level measures and implementation methods for clinical practice improvement
515 North State Street
Chicago, IL 60654
(800) 621-8335
http://www.ama-assn.org

AQA (formerly Ambulatory Care Quality Alliance)
Collaborative with documents on measurement and implementation principles
http://www.aqaalliance.org

Physician Quality Reporting Initiative
Centers for Medicare and Medicaid Services
Measures and resources for data collection and reporting for Medicare reimbursement
7500 Security Boulevard
Baltimore, MD 21244
(410) 786–3000
http://www.cms.hhs.gov/pqri/

The Joint Commission
Hospital and ambulatory standards and measures for accreditation
One Renaissance Boulevard
Oakbrook Terrace, IL 60181
(630) 792-5000
http://www.jointcommission.org/

National Committee for Quality Assurance—Healthcare Effectiveness Data and Information Set (HEDIS)
Standards, specifications, and benchmarks for health plan and physician-level measurement
1100 13th Street NW, Suite 1000
Washington, DC 20005
(202) 955-3500
http://www.ncqa.org/

National Perinatal Information Center/
Quality Analytic Service
Hospital reports and benchmarks on financial, clinical, and quality indicators
255 Chapman Street, Suite 200
Providence, RI 02905
(401) 274-0650
http://www.npic.org/

National Quality Forum
Consensus-developed endorsement organization of national measures and standards
601 13th Street NW, Suite 500 North
Washington, DC 20005
(202) 783-1300
http://www.qualityforum.org/

QualityNet
CMS-approved web site for resources and data reporting tools and applications for various health care settings
http://www.qualitynet.org/

APPENDIX D

National Organizations Involved in Performance Measurement

Name	Primary Role	Governance and Major Participants
Agency for Healthcare Research and Quality (AHRQ)	AHRQ sponsors and conducts research that provides evidence-based information on health care outcomes; quality; and cost, use, and access. The information helps health care decision makers—patients and clinicians, health system leaders, purchasers, and policymakers—make more informed decisions and improve the quality of health care services.	A Public Health Service agency in the U.S. Department of Health and Human Services (DHHS). Reporting to the DHHS Secretary, the Agency was authorized in 1989 as the Agency for Health Care Policy and Research and reauthorized in 1999 as AHRQ.

Major Quality Measurement Activities	Source of Core Funding
• The National Healthcare Quality Report (NHQR) is the first comprehensive national effort to measure the quality of health care in America. It includes a broad set of performance measures that can serve as baseline views of the quality of health care and presents data on services for seven clinical conditions: cancer, diabetes, end-stage renal disease, heart disease, HIV/AIDS, mental health, and respiratory disease. Also included are data on maternal and child health, nursing home and home health care, and patient safety.	Federal

- The National Healthcare Quality Report (NHQR) is the first comprehensive national effort to measure the quality of health care in America. It includes a broad set of performance measures that can serve as baseline views of the quality of health care and presents data on services for seven clinical conditions: cancer, diabetes, end-stage renal disease, heart disease, HIV/AIDS, mental health, and respiratory disease. Also included are data on maternal and child health, nursing home and home health care, and patient safety.
- The National Healthcare Disparities Report (NHDR), companion to the NHQR, provides measures of differences in access and use of health care services by various populations (divided by race and ethnicity, income, education, and insurance status where applicable) for all areas covered in the NHQR.
- The Consumer Assessment of Healthcare Providers and Systems (CAHPS) family of surveys is used by many public and private purchasers, including the National Committee for Quality Assurance (NCQA), to 1) develop and test questionnaires assessing health plans and services, 2) produce easily understandable reports communicate survey information to consumers, and 3) evaluate the usefulness of these reports for consumers in selecting health care plans and services.
- The National Quality Measures Clearinghouse™ houses the most current evidence-based quality measures and measure sets to evaluate and improve the quality of health care.
- The National Guidelines Clearinghouse™ contains evidence-based clinical practice guidelines that are often linked to measures.
- QualityTools (www.qualitytools.ahrq.gov) house the NHQR and the NHDR.
- The Prevention Quality Indicators* are a set of 16 measures that can be used with hospital inpatient discharge data to identify "ambulatory care sensitive conditions" for which good outpatient care can potentially prevent the need for hospitalization, or for which early intervention can prevent complications or more severe disease. They measure the outcomes of preventive and outpatient care through analysis of inpatient discharge data.
- The Inpatient Quality Indicators* consist of a set of 30 measures that reflect the quality of care inside hospitals and include inpatient mortality; utilization of procedures for which there are questions of overuse, underuse, or misuse; and volume of procedures for which there is evidence that a higher volume of procedures is associated with lower mortality.
- The Patient Safety Indicators* are a set of 29 measures that provide a perspective on patient safety by screening for problems that patients experience as a result of exposure to the health care system and that are likely amenable to prevention by changes at the system or provider level. (www.qualityindicators.ahrq.gov)

*The AHRQ Quality Indicators initially were developed as metrics for quality improvement; however, their use has evolved over time to include public reporting and pay for performance.

Name	Primary Role	Governance and Major Participants
Ambulatory Care Quality Alliance (AQA)	AQA is a collaborative effort initially convened by AHRQ, the American Academy of Family Physicians, the American College of Physicians, and America's Health Insurance Plans. The steering group has been expanded to include the American Medical Association, the American Osteopathic Association, the American College of Surgeons, the Society of Thoracic Surgeons, AARP, the National Partnership for Women and Families, and the Pacific Business Group on Health. Their mission is to improve health care quality and patient safety through a collaborative process in which key stakeholders agree on a strategy for measuring performance at the physician level; collecting and aggregating data in the least burdensome way; and reporting meaningful information to consumers, physicians, and other stakeholders to inform choices and improve outcomes.	Public–private partnership. The AQA consists of a large body of stakeholders that represents clinicians, consumers, purchasers, health plans, and others. Major participants: **Health care organizations:** ACP, AAFP, AMA, AMA Consortium, American Board of Internal Medicine, American Board of Medical Specialties, ACC, AAP, AAAAI, AOA, ACS, STS, MGMA, AHA, AAMC and state medical societies. **Private participants:** AARP, AFL-CIO, Consumer/ Purchaser Disclosure Project, Employer Health Care Alliance Corp., Leapfrog Group, General Motors, National Business Group on Health, National Business Coalition on Health, Pacific Business Group on Health, Medstat, Motorola, UPS, BellSouth, Xerox, and Marriott. **Public purchasers and other government agencies:** CMS, OPM, AHRQ, and Department of Treasury. **Health insurance plans:** Aetna, Anthem, Cigna, Health Net, Health Partners, Humana, Independence BCBS, Kaiser Permanente, Pacificare, Presbyterian Health Plan, Regence BCBS, UnitedHealth Group, Wellchoice, Harvard Pilgrim HealthCare, AHIP, Blue Cross Blue Shield Association. **Accrediting organizations:** NCQA, JCAHO, and URAC.
Centers for Medicare and Medicaid Services (CMS)	The federal agency responsible for administering Medicare, Medicaid, State Children's Health Insurance Program (SCHIP), Health Insurance Portability and Accountability Act (HIPPA), Clinical Laboratory Improvement Amendments (CLIA), and several other health-related programs. Their mission is to ensure health care security for beneficiaries.	An agency of DHHS. On July 1, 2001, the Health Care Financing Administration (HCFA) became CMS.

Major Quality Measurement Activities	Source of Core Funding
• Endorsed key parameters (criteria) for selecting performance measures. For example, evidence-based; clinical importance; scientific validity; feasibility; and relevance to physician performance, consumers, and purchasers.	Combination of federal and private
• Endorsed a standardized set of 26 measures for physician practices that draws heavily on the 2004 ambulatory care clinical performance measure set released by the AMA Consortium, CMS, and NCQA.	
• Expanding the initial "starter" set of measures to include specialty and subspecialty care measures, efficiency measures, and patient experience measures.	
• Working with CMS and AHRQ to finalize pilot projects that would utilize the endorsed measurement set and combine public and private payer data.	
• *Technical assistance:* Under the Quality Improvement Organization (QIO) program, CMS contracts with independent medical organizations to ensure the quality of medical care paid under the Medicare program to Medicare Advantage and fee-for-service beneficiaries.	Federal
• *Measure development:* CMS has collaborated with many organizations such as JCAHO, AQA, and HQA to develop measures in nursing homes, home health agencies, hospitals, dialysis facilities, and physician offices.	
• *Public reporting:* Web-based tools, such as the Nursing Home Compare, Home Health Compare, and Hospital Compare, that allow the public to compare data on the quality of providers were developed by CMS in collaboration with others.	
• *Financial incentives linked to quality:* CMS is conducting quality incentive demonstrations by awarding bonus payments to providers for high performance, most notably through the Premier Hospital Quality Incentive Demonstration and Physician Group Practice Demonstration. The Medicare Health Support Program is a pilot program under way addressing chronic care disease management for fee-for-service beneficiaries. In addition, hospitals are provided with financial incentive to report on performance measures through MMA 501(b).	

Name	Primary Role	Governance and Major Participants
Hospital Quality Alliance (HQA)	The purpose of the HQA initiative is to make information about hospital performance accessible to the public and to inform and invigorate efforts to improve quality. Voluntary reporting is essential to the success of this initiative.	Public–private partnership of hospitals, government agencies, quality experts, purchasers, consumer groups, and other health care organizations. These organizations have joined together to develop a shared national strategy for hospital quality measurement and are committed to advancing quality of care. Major participants: • American Hospital Association • Association of American Medical Colleges • Federation of American Hospitals • AARP • AFL-CIO • CMS • AHRQ • JCAHO • AMA • NQF • Consumer-Purchaser Disclosure Project
Joint Commission on Accreditation of Health-care Organizations (JCAHO)	JCAHO evaluates and accredits more than 15,000 health care organizations and programs in the United States. Its mission is to continuously improve the safety and quality of care provided to the public.	Private nonprofit. Governed by a 29-member Board of Commissioners that includes nurses, physicians, consumers, health care executives, purchasers, labor representatives, quality experts, ethicists, and educators. Major participants: • Commonwealth Fund • California Endowment • Robert Wood Johnson Foundation • AHRQ
Leapfrog Group	The Leapfrog Group is a voluntary initiative to mobilize employer purchasing power to improve the safety, quality, and affordability of health care for Americans. Their mission is to trigger leaps forward by supporting informed health care decisions by those who use and pay for health care, and to promote high-value health care through incentives.	Private. The Leapfrog Group includes over 170 members from a growing consortium of Fortune 500 companies and other large private and public health care purchasers that provide health benefits to more than 34 million Americans in all 50 states. Major participants: • Business Roundtable • Robert Wood Johnson Foundation
National Committee for Quality Assurance (NCQA)	NCQA is dedicated to improving health care quality through evaluation of health care at various levels of the system from health plans to medical groups and individual doctors. NCQA's mission is to transform health care through measurement, transparency, and accountability.	Private nonprofit. Advised by a board of directors, NCQA frequently works with the federal and state governments to advance shared goals. Major participants: • AHRQ • American Diabetes Association • American Heart Association/American Stroke Association • Bridges to Excellence • California Endowment Foundation • California HealthCare Foundation • Integrated Healthcare Association • Commonwealth Fund • Robert Wood Johnson Foundation • Bristol-Myers Squib • Pfizer

Major Quality Measurement Activities	Source of Core Funding
• Currently has 20 hospital quality measures. • Hospital Compare is a tool patients can use in making care decisions by providing the public with useful information on hospital quality of care in an easily accessible way. • HCAHPS—measuring patient perspectives on hospital care—and anticipated for public reporting in 2007.	Combination of federal and private
• In February 1997, the Joint Commission launched its ORYX® initiative, to develop evidence-based performance measures and integrate outcomes and other performance measurement data into the accreditation process. • In July 2002, hospitals began collecting core measure data on four initial core measurement areas: acute myocardial infarction; heart failure; community-acquired pneumonia; and pregnancy and related conditions • In January 2003, hospitals began transmitting their measurement results to the Joint Commission. • In 2004, surgical infection prevention measures were added as a data collection and submission option.	Combination of federal and private
• The Leapfrog Group identified and has since refined four hospital quality and safety practices that are the focus of its health care provider performance comparisons and hospital recognition and reward. All of the practices are endorsed by the National Quality Forum. Based on independent scientific evidence, the quality practices are: computer physician order entry, evidence-based hospital referral, intensive care unit (ICU) staffing by physicians experienced in critical care medicine, and the Leapfrog Safe Practices Score.	Private
• The Research group engages in collaborative research that explores new approaches to measuring and reporting on the quality and efficiency of health care. • The Analysis group provides both day-to-day analysis of NCQA Accreditation, Health Plan Employer Data and Information Set (HEDIS) and CAHPS databases, and design and analysis of statistical processes used in research projects and measure development and maintenance. • The Measures Development (or Quality Measurement) group is devoted to the development and maintenance of measures in HEDIS. • Working with the American Diabetes Association and the American Heart Association/American Stroke Association, established the Diabetes Physician Recognition program and the Heart/Stroke Physician Recognition program to identify physicians who demonstrate high quality care in these areas. • Developed Physician Practice Connections, a recognition program based on an evaluation of the presence and use of systems in office practice. • All three recognition programs have been adopted for use in pay for performance programs.	Combination of public and private

Name	Primary Role	Governance and Major Participants
National Quality Forum (NQF)	Established consequent to a Presidential Commission, the NQF was created primarily to standardize national performance measures, quality indicators, and similar metrics for health care. It was envisioned to be the singular body performing this function. Other functions envisioned for the NQF were to develop and implement a national strategy for health care quality measurement and reporting and to be an "honest-broker" convener for health care quality matters. The mission of the NQF is to improve American health care through endorsement of consensus-based national standards for measurement and public reporting of health care performance data that provide meaningful information about whether care is safe, timely, beneficial, patient-centered, equitable, and efficient.	Not-for-profit membership organization. Unique public–private partnership. About 300 member organizations. NQF is governed by a 29-member Board of Directors representing health care providers, health plans, consumers, purchasers, accreditors, researchers, and quality improvement organizations. Government members of the Board include CMS, AHRQ, VHA, ONCHIT, and NIH. Board also includes JCAHO, NCQA, IOM, AARP, GM, Physician Consortium for Performance Improvement, and elected representatives of the 4 Member Councils. Major participants: • AARP • Leapfrog Group, GM, Ford • 20 largest hospital organizations • CMS • AHRQ • VA • AMA, AAFP, medical specialty societies • National Partnership for Women and Children • Kaiser Permanente • Robert Wood Johnson Foundation
The Physician Consortium for Performance Improvement convened by the American Medical Association (AMA)	The Physician Consortium for Performance Improvement's (the Consortium) mission is to improve patient health and safety by 1) identifying and developing evidence-based clinical performance measures, 2) promoting implementation of effective and relevant clinical performance improvement activities, and 3) advancing the science of clinical performance measurement and improvement.	Professional societies. The Consortium is currently formalizing its governance and structure. The Consortium includes physicians and experts in methodology convened by the AMA. The Consortium includes representatives from more than 70 national medical specialty and state medical societies, the AHRQ, CMS, and others. Representatives from employers, health plans, and consumer groups participate in measure development work groups.

Major Quality Measurement Activities	Source of Core Funding
• Over 200 national consensus standards have been endorsed so far for care settings across the continuum of care (eg, acute care hospitals, ambulatory care, nursing homes, home care, palliative and hospice care, other) as well as for conditions (eg, cancer, asthma, acute coronary syndrome, diabetes, and deep vein thrombosis) and issues (eg, patient safety, reportable events, medication use). A variety of workshops have been conducted to address specific issues related to quality.	Membership dues, contracts and grants, and a combination of federal and private funding.
• The Consortium selects topics for performance measures development that are actionable, for which established clinical recommendations are available, and for which feasible data sources exist. Work groups review the levels of evidence provided in clinical practice guidelines that demonstrate potential positive impact on health outcomes and propose feasible measures for inclusion in a physician performance measurement set. All specifications for Consortium measures are available at www.physicianconsortium.org, including specifications for electronic health record systems. • As of October 2005, 24 Consortium measures have been NQF-endorsed, and several are included in the AQA starter set.	AMA. In-kind funding and national medical specialty societies. Additional funding for measure development from contracts with CMS.

Reprinted with permission from Performance Measurement: Accelerating Improvement, 2006, by the National Academy of Sciences, Washington, DC.

APPENDIX E

World Health Organization
Surgical Safety Checklist

Surgical Safety Checklist

Before induction of anaesthesia	Before skin incision	Before patient leaves operating room
(with at least nurse and anaesthetist)	(with nurse, anaesthetist and surgeon)	(with nurse, anaesthetist and surgeon)

Before induction of anaesthesia

Has the patient confirmed his/her identity, site, procedure, and consent?
☐ Yes

Is the site marked?
☐ Yes
☐ Not applicable

Is the anaesthesia machine and medication check complete?
☐ Yes

Is the pulse oximeter on the patient and functioning?
☐ Yes

Does the patient have a:

Known allergy?
☐ No
☐ Yes

Difficult airway or aspiration risk?
☐ No
☐ Yes, and equipment/assistance available

Risk of >500ml blood loss (7ml/kg in children)?
☐ No
☐ Yes, and two IVs/central access and fluids planned

Before skin incision

☐ Confirm all team members have introduced themselves by name and role.

☐ Confirm the patient's name, procedure, and where the incision will be made.

Has antibiotic prophylaxis been given within the last 60 minutes?
☐ Yes
☐ Not applicable

Anticipated Critical Events

To Surgeon:
☐ What are the critical or non-routine steps?
☐ How long will the case take?
☐ What is the anticipated blood loss?

To Anaesthetist:
☐ Are there any patient-specific concerns?

To Nursing Team:
☐ Has sterility (including indicator results) been confirmed?
☐ Are there equipment issues or any concerns?

Is essential imaging displayed?
☐ Yes
☐ Not applicable

Before patient leaves operating room

Nurse Verbally Confirms:
☐ The name of the procedure
☐ Completion of instrument, sponge and needle counts
☐ Specimen labelling (read specimen labels aloud, including patient name)
☐ Whether there are any equipment problems to be addressed

To Surgeon, Anaesthetist and Nurse:
☐ What are the key concerns for recovery and management of this patient?

This checklist is not intended to be comprehensive. Additions and modifications to fit local practice are encouraged. Revised 1/2009.

Checklist for Surgical Safety, World Health Organization 2009. Available at http://whqlibdoc.who.int/publications/2009/9789241598590_eng_checklist.pdf. Reprinted with permission.

APPENDIX F

Sample Application for Privileges: Department of Obstetrics and Gynecology

This sample application for privileges is provided for educational purposes only.
It may require modification for use in a particular facility.

1. Name:_____

2. Department to which I am applying: _____

3. Other department(s) in which clinical privileges are held or sought: _____

_____

4. Subject to consultation requirements and other policies, I understand that in exercising my clinical privileges granted, I am constrained by relevant hospital policies requiring consultations for difficult diagnoses, conditions of extreme severity, and procedures and conditions that are beyond my area of training, specialization, and current competence and experience; by hospital policies concerning types of patients for whom it does not have appropriate resources (facilities, equipment, or personnel) to treat except on an emergency basis; and by such special policies as may from time to time be adopted.

5. Emergency situations:

   I also understand

   (a) that the privileges are being requested for regular use in my practice;

   (b) that it is not necessary to request emergency clinical privileges;

   (c) that an emergency is deemed to exist whenever serious permanent harm or aggravation of injury or disease is imminent, or the life of a patient is in immediate danger, and any delay in administering treatment could add danger;

   (d) that in such emergency, when better alternative sources of care are not reasonably available given the patient's condition, I am authorized and will be assisted to do everything possible to save the patient's life or to save the patient from serious harm to the degree permitted by my license but regardless of department affiliation or privileges;

   (e) and that if I provide services to a patient in an emergency, I am obligated to use appropriate consultative assistance when available and to arrange, when it is my responsibility, for appropriate follow-up care.

General Provisions

Basis for Granting Privileges

1. Applicants requesting clinical privileges must demonstrate satisfactory training, experience, and current competence for the privileges being requested and must agree to comply with the provisions contained in the medical staff bylaws.

2. Each applicant requesting privileges in the department of obstetrics and gynecology should be required to present his or her application and a list of recent cases for review by the department chief.

(For physicians who have just completed an ob-gyn residency program, the list could be the senior resident case list.) When family physicians or nurse–midwives request privileges, an equivalent list of recently managed cases, representing the full range of privileges being requested, must also be submitted.

Provisional Period

1. All new appointees to the department of obstetrics and gynecology must undergo a minimum provisional period of no less than 12 months. The

practitioner should have admitted a minimum number of cases to the hospital, completed an equivalent number of surgical procedures, or both, as defined by the institution.

2. At the chair's discretion, any additional documentation deemed necessary to assess an applicant's competency in specific procedures during the provisional period may be requested. This documentation may include evidence of specific education or training in a procedure either during residency training or through postresidency courses.

3. At the conclusion of their provisional period, those individuals who did not meet the minimum criteria stipulated under Number 1, or those who requested other than active staff status, should provide the chair with a detailed listing of each case completed within the department as well as the description, scope, and breadth of their practice at other institutions. In addition to the hospital's quality improvement review, the department chair also may request information from other institutions where the individual practices to assess overall competency for the procedure(s) requested.

4. Those individuals requesting privileges for a new procedure must have successfully completed their initial provisional period and have been appointed to the medical staff without restriction.

    They also should submit evidence they have completed an educational or training program in the specific procedure either in a residency program or through postgraduate residency training. In addition, each applicant should submit a letter from the director of a residency program stating that he or she is competent in the respective procedure and has completed the appropriate training.

Individuals requesting privileges for a new procedure must be deemed competent to perform the procedure by an individual currently credentialed for that procedure in the department. However, if this is the first time these privileges have been requested within the department, arrangements should be made to ensure that the applicant is adequately evaluated before granting full, unrestricted privileges. In general, a minimum number of cases with preceptorship or observation, as defined by the institution, are required before full, unrestricted privileges can be granted for a new procedure.

New, Untried, Unproved, or Experimental Procedures and Treatment Modalities and Instrumentation

Experimental drugs, procedures, or other therapies or tests may be administered or performed only after approval of protocols involved by the committee responsible for the institutional review board function. Any other new, untried, or unproved procedure or treatment modality or instrumentation may be performed or used only after the regular credentialing process has been completed, and the privilege to perform or use said procedure or treatment modality or instrument has been granted to an individual practitioner. For the purposes of this paragraph, a new, untried, or unproved procedure or treatment modality or instrumentation is one that is not generalizable from an established procedure or treatment modality or instrumentation involving the same or similar skills, the same or similar instrumentation and technique, the same or similar complications, or the same or similar indications as the established procedure or treatment modality or instrumentation.

APPENDIX G

Report of the Presidential Task Force on Patient Safety in the Office Setting

Task Force Charge

To assist, inform, and enable Fellows to design and implement processes that will facilitate a safe and effective environment for the more invasive technologies currently being introduced into the office setting.

Introduction

Patient safety includes activities designed to eliminate or mitigate any harm that could occur during the entire time that a patient remains in the care of a health care provider. Increased attention by educational and regulatory organizations has effectively elevated patient safety activities into the consciousness of all parties and stakeholders, including patients.

This task force seeks to reinvigorate the attention of clinicians on patient safety activities in the office setting. This practice setting has traditionally served as the home base for health care providers. An increasing number of invasive and potentially harmful procedures are migrating from the more highly regulated surgery center or hospital surgery units into the office setting. Regulation of office surgical procedures may be nonexistent, difficult to enforce, or resisted by the physician. It should be obvious, however, that once a patient has been invited into this office setting they have the right to expect the same level of patient safety that occurs in the more regulated hospital setting. Health care providers should expect some regulation and seek the help of all stakeholders to assist in establishing a safe, transparent environment for health care delivery. Major elements of office setting safety include effective communication, staff competency, medication error avoidance, accurate patient tracking mechanisms, anesthesia safety, and general procedural safety. Although all of these elements are important, the primary focus of this task force is on providing information and tools to create a safe environment for the introduction of invasive technologies into the office setting. The task force's highest priority is to assist Fellows in establishing physician and staff competency within an office setting. In this document, we will define the office level according to the depth of anesthesia:

> Level I—Local anesthesia with minimal preoperative oral anxiolytic medication
>
> Level II—Moderate sedation
>
> Level III—Deep sedation or general anesthesia

Rather than creating a finished product that may not apply in all individual office settings, we suggest integrating a patient safety culture into every standing committee, every agenda, and every educational opportunity provided to Fellows. This will allow for customization of safety policies, procedures, and practices in any office setting.

It is now well recognized that due to patient, physician, and payer preferences more invasive procedures will continue to move from the hospital operating room into an office setting. This trend creates the need for more robust and effective patient safety initiatives in the office. Establishing a safe environment for patient care in the office setting will require additional effort, expense, and training. On the other hand, these initiatives will be cost-effective by reducing the expense of correcting errors, increasing efficiency, and improving patient satisfaction.

Office Medical Director

Any facility performing outpatient surgical procedures should have a designated medical director. Similar to a movie director, the office medical director has the responsibility to verify that all participants are qualified and cognizant of their roles. They should assure that the set is prepared properly for any given performance. This requires teamwork from all participants: the receptionist, nursing staff, physicians, midlevel providers, and outside participants such as laboratory, pathology, and vendor services. In a solo practice, the physician should assume the role of medical director. In a group practice, one of the partners should be designated as medical director.

In very large practices, other individuals may assume some of the responsibilities listed below (eg, Director of Quality Assurance). The medical director verifies the qualifications and safety of people, equipment, space, and supplies which requires a full understanding of all elements necessary for the safe completion of a planned procedure. This document outlines many elements vital for safe practices; medical directors should familiarize themselves not only with the content of this document but also should expect to adapt the information and tools to their own needs. Holding regular team meetings and involving the collective efforts of all stakeholders should help ensure a safe environment for the performance of invasive procedures.

Checklists and drills are two vital tools assisting the medical director to ensure the safe practice of invasive procedures. In the next section, examples of both will be provided and each practice may modify the examples according to their unique clinical circumstances. Checklists with a box checked to verify completion of each step should be filled out for each procedure. This checklist format is used in the aviation industry for routine as well as emergency procedures. Emergency drills are done at least quarterly, so people can apply common sense, know their roles, complete their tasks, and not panic during a true emergency.

Checklists

(Italicized bullets are expanded upon further in the document.)

Office Set-Up Checklist

- *Comply with policy and procedure manual* (updated with the College's current *Guidelines for Women's Health Care*)
- *Provide patients' rights handout*
- *Provide informed consent materials and sign forms*
- Arrange for transfer agreement with nearby hospital
- Assure adequate equipment for level of anesthesia and analgesia, examples include:
  - Blood pressure and P/heart rate monitor
  - Pulse oximeter
  - Exhaled carbon dioxide monitoring for deep sedation
  - Reliable oxygen source
  - Suction
  - Resuscitation equipment including defibrillator
  - Cardiac monitor
  - Auxiliary electrical power source
  - Emergency medication

- Maintain, test, and inspect all equipment per manufacturer's recommendations
- *Ability to monitor level of sedation (see Anesthesia)*
- *Ability to rescue patient from excessive sedation (see Anesthesia)*
- *Quarterly mock drill*
- Compliance with state board of pharmacy and Drug Enforcement Administration
- Compliance with local building codes, fire codes, and the Occupational Safety and Health Administration
- Compliance with state and professional guidelines
- An Advanced Cardiac Life Support (ACLS), Pediatric Advanced Life Support (PALS), or Basic Life Support (BLS) certified physician or other health care professional immediately available to provide emergency resuscitation
- *Assure that an office-based surgery procedure record is available*
- *Adverse event reporting system*
- *Procedure outcome reporting system in place*
- *Credentialing and privileging of participating providers*

Preoperative Checklist

- *Meets office-based surgery requirements*
- *Meets American Society of Anesthesiologists (ASA) Physical Status I criteria or medically controlled ASA Physical Status II*
- Prescreening verification that the patient is a candidate for an office-based procedure. Contraindications include but are not limited to:
  - Personal or family history of adverse reaction to local anesthetic
  - History of previous failure with local anesthesia or low pain threshold
  - An acute respiratory process
  - Failure to comply with preoperative dietary restrictions
  - Substance abuse
  - High-risk airway assessment
  - Abnormal blood sugars
  - Pregnancy (unless procedure is pregnancy related)
- Document appropriate workup, patient selection, and informed consent
- No change in medical condition since previous office visit
- Preoperative vital signs
- *Current history and physical*
- Review and record all medications taken previously that day

- Confirm *nil per os* (nothing by mouth—NPO) status
- Confirm preoperative instructions followed
- Review allergies
- Confirm patient has an escort driver
- Document no change in patient's medical condition
- Confirm presence of any indicated lab work (eg, glucose level in a diabetic)

Intraoperative Checklist

- *Time-out* (verify provider, patient, surgical site, and procedure)
- Record intraoperative medications
- If sedation implemented, monitor and document oxygen saturation, blood pressure, pulse, and level of alertness every 5 minutes
- For hysteroscopic procedures, record cavity assessment per manufacturer's guidelines

Postoperative Checklist

- Record vital signs and ensure return to within 20% of baseline
- Document adequate level of consciousness, pain control, ability to tolerate liquids by mouth, and ability to void (if appropriate for the procedure)
- Discharge instruction sheet that includes how to recognize a postoperative emergency and steps to follow should one occur after discharge (eg, hemorrhage)
- Postoperative follow-up call within 48 hours
- Schedule appropriate postoperative follow-up appointment
- Record long-term outcome
- Record complications

Mock Drills

Drills should be conducted quarterly based on possible complications to ensure that all staff members are knowledgeable about their roles. For each drill all staff should be present (others such as front desk personnel are important and would have a role to call 911 or arrange for additional help), and their role should be clearly defined. Examples of mock drills included in this document can be used as templates to practice everyone's response in the event of unanticipated complications. Mock drills are a powerful way to ensure that all members of a patient care team are coordinated in the care of that patient. Each drill can be accomplished quickly. It is effective to have a team member role play a patient and act out the drills to help the entire team

accomplish the goal of handling a potential complication in a standard, step-by-step manner. There should be a debriefing following a drill to review what was done well and what could be improved next time.

Drills should be based on critical or frequent complications, resuscitation, or nonclinical situations (eg, intimate partner violence or environmental disaster). Drills should focus on individual roles and include the following responsibilities specific to each person:

- Communication
  - Call for help (within the office)
  - Notify front desk about incident
  - Front desk should prepare to dial 911 if necessary and wait for ambulance at entrance of building if 911 is called
  - Verbally confirm roles with others ("I will call 911" or "I will go wait outside")
  - Communicate situation with other patients or family members
  - Debrief with all office staff after patient recovers
- Interventions (dependent on the situation)
  - Place patient in supine position and elevate legs
  - Open and support airway
  - Check for pulse and blood pressure
  - Give fluids as tolerated

See Appendix G-1 for specific examples of drills that may be implemented.

Policy and Procedure Manual

The office manual should include all policies and procedures pertaining to office-based surgery.

Informed Consent

Informed consent is a process, not a signed form. Ultimately, the operating physician is responsible for assuring that the patient fully understands the risks and benefits of the proposed procedure as well as alternatives. In addition to discussing the specifics of the procedure in the case of surgery in the office setting, there should also be a discussion about the risks and benefits of performing the procedure in the office versus an ambulatory surgery center or hospital.

Written and audiovisual materials may be used as well as a discussion with a nurse or medical assistant to facilitate the patient's understanding. However, final consent for the procedure and the location must be a shared decision between the physician and the patient.

An additional element of informed consent focuses on the partnership between the patient and the health care provider. These principles should be integrated into the informed consent process.

Patient Rights

Ideally, a practice should inform all patients of their rights and responsibilities. As part of any informed consent for the provision of general care or treatment, many practices include a patient bill of rights.

In the accreditation process of virtually every ambulatory health care facility, the surveyor looks for a written patient's bill of rights including a corresponding list of patient responsibilities. These two documents should clearly inform patients of every right they can enjoy in the practice, as well as what the practice should expect from the patient.

Typical rights of patients include, but are not limited to, the right to:

- Privacy
- Being treated with dignity and respect
- Confidentiality of patient records
- Complete medical information about the patient's condition, prognosis, and treatment options
- Participation in decisions about care
- Fees and payment policies
- Access to services at the practice
- Any advance directive policies of the practice (especially if the practice chooses to not honor them)
- Information about the credentials of their health care providers

Typical patient responsibilities include, but are not limited to:

- Being honest and accurate when providing medical history information and information about the use of any medications, over-the-counter products, allergies, or sensitivities
- Following the treatment plan of the health care provider
- Informing the health care provider of any living will or medical power of attorney that might affect the patient's care
- Being responsible for any charges not covered by insurance
- Being respectful of the health care provider and staff

See Appendix G-2 for an example.

Anesthesia

The type and level of anesthesia should be dictated by the procedure with input based on patient preference.

The decision regarding type of anesthesia should not be altered based on limitations of equipment or personnel in the office setting. Such limitations might necessitate performing the procedure in a more acute care facility. The level of anesthesia (light, moderate, or deep sedation or general anesthesia) will dictate the equipment and personnel needed.

All necessary medication should be in the room and immediately available before the onset of the procedure. Controlled drugs should be logged out from a secure location. A medication administration log (including the use of local anesthetic agents) must be maintained during the procedure.

A person responsible for administration of medication and monitoring the patient must be present in the procedure room. Depending on the level of anesthesia, this monitoring function might be assumed by a medical assistant, nurse, certified nurse anesthetist, or anesthesiologist. In all but the last case, these individuals must work under protocols with the surgeon assuming responsibility. Physicians administering or supervising moderate sedation or analgesia, deep sedation or analgesia, or general anesthesia should have appropriate education and training.

There should be a designated recovery area adequately staffed and equipped to assure that the patient has the level of monitoring appropriate for the procedure and anesthesia. For all but light (Level I) sedation, there should be oxygen and suction available.

If it is anticipated that any level of sedation may be needed, staff must confirm that the patient has an escort to drive the patient home before starting the procedure. No patient should leave the office following any level of sedation without an escort.

Please note the level of anesthesia achieved is the primary concern regarding patient safety and not the agents used (ie, oral versus intravenous medications). Whether given orally or parenterally, narcotics and sedatives pose similar risks. The patient should be evaluated for depth of sedation regardless of mode of delivery, including all the recommended monitoring equipment and procedures. Please refer to Appendix G-3 regarding the levels of sedation and anesthesia from the ASA.

In addition, a collaborative practice integrating gynecologic surgeons and anesthesiologists may emerge given the increasing migration of more complex invasive procedures to the office setting.

Procedure Outcome Reporting System

Continuous quality assessment and improvement is vital to assure the professionalism of the office and safety of the patient. A designated individual must be responsible for this activity. This might be the duty of the medical director or in large offices it could be another individual.

A log should be maintained to evaluate processes as well as outcomes. Examples of measures are in part specific to the procedure and might include equipment malfunction, compliance with checklists, adequacy of anesthesia and postoperative analgesia, and maintenance of sterile technique.

Outcome measures should include intraoperative and postoperative complications as well as infection. Patient satisfaction is also an important outcome measure that may give insight to areas for improvement. The patient should be called one to two days following the procedure to assess for delayed complications. In addition, at that time the patient can be asked questions regarding satisfaction with the office personnel and procedures, wait times, and if the patient's outcome and recovery met expectations. Ideally this call should be made by a trusted member of the health care team experienced in patient advocacy, such as a nurse or physician's assistant. Patient satisfaction can also be assessed by a survey filled out at the time of the postoperative appointment.

All significant complications should be carefully analyzed by a multidisciplinary team to determine and remediate any latent system errors.

Results of these quality assessment measures should be recorded and periodically reviewed (monthly or quarterly based on the volume of activity) to evaluate trends that may suggest potential areas for improvement. A plan for improvement should be discussed and implemented, with the results tracked to be certain the problem has been adequately addressed.

Ability to Rescue Patient from Excessive Sedation, Emergency Medication, and Resuscitative Policy

These policies should be based on the ASA levels or other scale according to level of invasiveness.

1. Level I—Personnel with training in BLS should be immediately available until all patients are discharged home. Emergency equipment for cardiorespiratory support and treatment of anaphylaxis must be readily available (and in good working order) for those who are trained to use it.

2. Level II—A minimum of two staff persons must be on the premises, one of whom shall be a licensed physician and surgeon and a licensed health care professional with current training in advanced resuscitative techniques (eg, ACLS, PALS) until all patients are discharged home. Additionally, at least one physician must be present or immediately available any time patients are present. Emergency equipment, ACLS medication and trained personnel for cardio-respiratory support and treatment of anaphylaxis must be immediately available.

Time-Outs

Upon arrival to the office, each patient should provide:

1. Photo identification
2. Relevant insurance information
3. Relevant medical information

Immediately prior to beginning the procedure or administering any anesthesia, a time-out must be observed allowing each member of the medical team to verify:

1. That all relevant documents, imaging results, and lab tests have been reviewed and are consistent with each other
2. That all team members and the patient agree on the procedure to be performed and the exact location for it to be performed
3. That the incision site is marked in a way visible even after the patient is prepped and draped (as indicated by the specific procedure)
4. That this is the
   a. Correct patient (using two independent identifiers)
   b. Correct procedure
   c. Correct site

Credentialing, Privileging, and Accreditation

The process of evaluating the competency to perform office-based procedures should be similar to the process followed for inpatient procedures. Physicians performing office-based procedures and the setting in which they will be performed should be subject to a system ensuring appropriate credentialing, privileging, and, in some cases, accreditation. Further, procedures initially performed solely in an inpatient setting should only be converted to the office setting after the provider has demonstrated competency in an accredited operating room setting.

Credentialing, privileging, and accreditation—though often used interchangeably and loosely—refer to three very distinct, though related, events. This section will define each of the terms and explain how they interrelate.

Credentialing

Essentially, credentialing involves verifying that people are indeed who they purport to be. It involves:

- Verification of education and training, including medical school, residency, board status, and any other work experience.
- Primary or secondary source verification: relevant schools, hospitals, and agencies can be contacted to verify if the license is in good standing and to

identify any history of disciplinary action. Verification also may rely on accepted secondary sources such as web sites of the American Medical Association (AMA) or even state health departments and national resources like the Office of the Inspector General.

- Ideally, the National Practitioner Data Bank (NPDB) should also be queried since employed or partner physicians may develop unknown claims especially from pre-employment activities.

- There is an ongoing need to recheck the data on a regular basis, usually every 1–3 years. Some items, such as previously verified medical school, residency, and training will not change. However, peer review information, the National Practitioner Data Bank, and liability claims in process may indeed change.

- A credentialing system also should require notification of any material changes in credentialed health care providers' status. For instance, if their privileges are limited at the hospital or surgical center, this must be reported to the practice too. Likewise, a health department investigation of a complaint resulting in anything other than full exculpation needs to be reported.

- Initial credentialing should include at least one or two peer letters of support, indicating perceived skill levels and competence.

- For recredentialing, it is not unreasonable to forgo outside peer assessments if the health care provider does enough activity for the practice's quality assurance and risk management system to oversee the quality of the health care provider's work. This ongoing peer review data should be considered in recredentialing decisions.

Although the foregoing process may appear onerous, many practices are already doing a lot of these tasks, on behalf of hospitals, surgical centers, and managed care companies. Applications for initial credentialing include some or all of the following:

- Copy of current state medical license
- Copy of current Drug Enforcement Administration certificate
- Copy of the current cover letter for liability insurance indicating limits of coverage
- Copy of current delineation of privileges from a local hospital
- Copy of board certification (if applicable)
- Copy of any special certificates held (eg, laser)
- Current curriculum vitae
- Letter of recommendation from the Chief of Surgery or Division Chief

- Letter of recommendation from a surgeon, in the same specialty, who holds staff privileges at the institution
- Signature sheets for institutional policies (eg, Health Insurance Portability and Accountability Act, compliance program, or patient safety)
- Any fees

Privileging

Once the process of credentialing is complete, the health care provider's specific role description must be agreed on by the practice. In small practices, the governing body may be the partners themselves. In larger practices, an executive committee or even a board of directors assumes the role of a governing body. The governing body is responsible for privileging—actually delineating the specific procedures each health care provider may perform. Procedures initially performed solely in an inpatient setting should only be converted to the office setting after the health care provider has demonstrated competency in an accredited operating room setting.

Typically, privileging should entail:

- Verification of specific training in certain areas (especially procedures and skills that may be newer and were acquired postresidency)
- Verifying actual competence in performing those procedures
- Specifying procedures allowed (ablation, loop electrosurgical excision procedures [LEEPs], dilatation and curettage [D&C] in detail)
- All procedures must be approved by the practice in order to perform them

A fairly complete list of procedures performed in the office might be found in a privileges list used in a local ambulatory surgery center or hospital outpatient department. See Appendix G-4 for sample forms.

Accreditation

Accreditation refers to the practice or facility. There are several accrediting agencies that can be utilized. The list includes the Accreditation Association for Ambulatory Health Care, the Joint Commission, and the American Association for Accreditation of Ambulatory Surgery Facilities, and several others accepted nationally as bona fide accrediting agencies.

A practice may seek accreditation for various reasons but generally there are internal and external indications to pursue it. Internally, the accreditation process involves and augments a self-assessment process that looks critically at the practice structure and function and provides important consultative advice on how to improve processes to enhance the quality of care provided.

Externally, it is a seal of approval from a recognized authority that the practice meets high quality standards. In an age of increasingly consumer-directed health decisions, having a certificate in a waiting room and on any marketing material will help direct savvy health consumers to the office. Also, with respect to contracting with insurers, an accredited organization may be eligible for an enhanced fee schedule or at least argue successfully against more onerous managed care requirements like precertification of certain procedures.

The steps for the usual accreditation process include the following:

- An accrediting organization is invited to survey a practice or facility, applying its published standards to all aspects of the practice.
- The practice's physical structure, ownership, and legal status are reviewed.
- Policies, procedures, protocols, governance, and overall compliance with its own policies and protocols are examined.

Generally, the surveyor's role is to evaluate systems, point out strengths, as well as opportunities for improvement, and consult on methods for improvement. Sometimes quality of care is excellent, but is not documented properly.

Interrelationship of Credentialing, Privileging, and Accreditation

How do these three activities interrelate with respect to performance of outpatient procedures in the office setting? To a large extent, many practices perform the credentialing and privileging already, albeit informally.

For instance, when new physicians are employed, they must be credentialed by any hospital and outpatient surgical facility in which they will work, and also privileged by those entities to be allowed to do certain procedures.

Most likely, each practice already maintains a file for each physician and other collaborative providers of care like certified nurse–midwives, physician assistants, and advanced practice registered nurses. Those files include a current copy of licenses, continuing medical education certificates, and any additional certificates verifying specialized training (eg, nuchal thickness ultrasound training, tension-free vaginal tape or transobturator tape training, or laser use training) obtained since residency was completed.

To begin internal credentialing and privileging for office procedures, the practice would essentially use this existing information. A formal application process not only credentials the health care providers but also allows them to apply for specific privileges. See a sample of delineation of privileges and a list of procedures in Appendix G-4 and a model application in Appendix F.

Credentials must be verified; this verification can be accomplished from secondary sources. There are web resources (AMA or state and federal websites) that verify if a license is in good standing as well as show any formal complaints or actions taken against any licensed individual. Verification of credentials can also be done through documented communication with the affiliated hospital's credentialing office.

Once credentialing is done, the practice must decide whether the health care provider can be privileged to perform specific procedures. The acceptance of credentials and granting of privileges must be done by the practice's governing body, which can be the partners in a meeting or the board of directors if it is formally organized. Either way, formal minutes should be kept to document the decision.

Simply put, credentialing verifies that physicians or other health care providers are indeed who they say they are. Formal education, training, licensure, and board certification are verified.

Privileging, on the other hand, is the granting of permission to perform specific procedures in the practice. This should be as inclusive as possible. For instance, endometrial biopsy, colposcopy, ultrasound, LEEPs, endometrial or laser ablations of the cervix, Bartholin's incision and drainage, and anything typically found on a hospital privileging list should be included if it is anticipated to be performed in the office.

Peer review should be included by soliciting peers' opinions of the applicant's competence and should at least be done upon initial application for privileges. If the reappointment process includes ongoing peer review in the practice itself (by tracking outcomes, near misses, or adverse events and watching for outliers) separately polling peers may not be necessary.

Accreditation is something more practices may seek in the future. Many states already require it if certain levels of anesthesia are used in the office or facility—typically moderate sedation or deeper anesthesia will trigger this requirement.

Patient Safety and the Relationship With Industry for Procedures Conducted in the Office Setting

Technology has provided opportunities for minimally invasive procedures to move into the office setting. This requires training of personnel and maintenance of durable equipment involved. Industry should create and sustain a culture of safety for procedures and equipment they develop. Many companies have recognized this need and provide resources to maintain patient safety. This should include but is not limited to the following areas:

1. Training of surgeons to include didactic training and proctoring

2. Assisting surgeons in office set-up including safety protocols for the use of equipment

3. Providing help in credentialing providers in specific techniques

4. Providing requirements for safety protocols of sufficient strength prior to placement of devices into the office

5. Training of support staff that may assist in running equipment

6. Periodic evaluation and maintenance of durable equipment above simple reliance on warranty

7. Providing data sheets for ongoing evaluation of outcomes and safe practices including "near misses"

8. Providing checklists specific to procedures and equipment that are standardized and focused on patient safety

9. Helping offices establish mock drills specific to their procedures and equipment

10. Notifying current users of best practices and improvements as they become available

11. Providing detailed patient information to include relevant preoperative and postoperative care specifics that focus not only on the procedure but attention on safety

Industry should partner with providers in providing a safe environment for these procedures rather than relying solely on the physician to take the full responsibility.

Conclusion

The Presidential Task Force on Patient Safety in the Office Setting convened to consider the effect of a changing health care environment with specific reference to the increase of invasive procedures performed in the office. This document should be viewed as an attempt to increase the awareness of Fellows of the American College of Obstetricians and Gynecologists in becoming vigilant at creating a culture of safety relating to office practice. It provides suggestions and educational opportunities for improvement but should not be viewed as a standard. The goal should be to create an environment to address the solutions to each specific practice. The medical director should counsel with colleagues and supportive staff to individualize their own adoption of these principles. Ultimately, all health care providers must incorporate patient safety in all aspects of office-based care.

APPENDIX G-1

Mock Drills

At least one of these drills should be conducted quarterly, possibly on a rotating basis. They are based on possible complications, and are to ensure that all staff members are knowledgeable about their role should a complication occur. For each drill, all staff who participate in office surgery should be present, and the roles for each aspect of patient care and safety should be clearly defined.

These examples of mock drills can be used as templates for a simulation of an event, which is a powerful tool to ensure that all members of a patient care team are coordinated in the care of that patient. Each drill can be accomplished quickly. It is effective to have a team member role play a patient and act out these drills to help the entire team accomplish the goal of handling a potential complication in a standard, stepwise fashion.

1. Vasovagal episode
2. Local anesthetic complication
3. Cardiac event (myocardial infarction)
4. Allergic reaction
5. Uterine hemorrhage
6. Respiratory arrest
7. Excessive sedation

Vasovagal Episode

Description: Syncope, or fainting, is usually a transient loss of consciousness that can be associated with anxiety, prolonged fasting and dehydration, or allergic reactions to medications or systemic injection of local anesthetics.

Signs and Symptoms:

- Dizziness, light-headed feeling
- Loss of consciousness
- Nausea, vomiting
- Weakness
- Cool, clammy, and pale skin
- Decreased blood pressure and pulse

Treatment:

- Place patient in supine position and elevate legs
- Open and support airway
- Check for pulse and blood pressure
- Give fluids as tolerated
- Assess for possible allergic reaction to medications or systemic administration of local anesthetic and act accordingly (ACLS)
- Assess for level of consciousness then reassure patient

Disposition:

- If the patient can slowly sit then stand without dizziness, she may be discharged and instructed to seek medical follow up.
- Consider evaluation to rule out cardiac or neurological basis if suspected.
- Administer CPR and call 911 if the patient has swelling, loss of consciousness, or convulsions associated with low blood pressure.

Approved by:_____ Date:_____

Local Anesthetic Toxicity Reaction

Description: Toxicity reactions occur when local anesthetic is injected into the circulatory system. This results in cardiac depression, possible convulsions, and can lead to cardiac and respiratory compromise.

Signs and Symptoms:

- Cardiac depression: low blood pressure, slow heart rate (initially a fast heart rate if local anesthetic has epinephrine in it)
- Ringing in ears, metallic taste in mouth

Treatment:

- Place patient in supine position and elevate legs

- Optimize airway with head extension and jaw thrust and give oxygen by bag mask
- Be prepared to treat convulsions
- Monitor oxygen saturation, blood pressure, carotid pulse or listen to heart
- Start basic life support and call 911 if there is no pulse or heart tone

Disposition:

- Minor toxicity reaction:
  - The patient may have minor symptoms with no cardiac compromise
  - Do not give any more local anesthetic
  - The patient will recover without further treatment
- Major toxicity reaction with convulsions or cardiac compromise:
  - Call 911 for assistance with IV, CPR, and transport

Approved by:_____ Date:_____

Myocardial Infarction

Description: Patients with partial blockage of the coronary arteries may experience heart pain or angina pectoris when blood flow to the heart muscle is restricted. Should blood flow to the heart muscle stop completely, muscle damage will result in a heart attack or myocardial infarction.

Signs and Symptoms:

- Pallor, nausea, vomiting
- Weak pulse with irregular rhythm
- Chest pain, arm pain, back pain, or no pain

Treatment:

- Supplemental oxygen
- Monitor electrocardiogram for arrhythmia
- Nitroglycerin, sublingual, one or two pills every five minutes until chest pain relieved or onset of a headache
- Aspirin unless contraindicated

Disposition:

- Call 911. The patient should not exert themselves in any way. They should be transported immediately to the hospital.

Approved by:_____ Date:_____

Allergic Reactions

Description: Severe allergic reactions to drugs are rare. These reactions occur when a patient is given a drug that stimulates the immune system. A tiny amount of the drug may cause a severe allergic reaction or anaphylaxis, which can cause cardiac and respiratory compromise.

Signs and Symptoms:

- Minor: rash, wheels, itching, swelling (face, hands)
- Major: wheezing, if severe can cause respiratory distress
- Hypotension—low blood pressure
- Oxygen desaturation
- Rapid pulse, rapid breathing

Treatment:

- Minor:
  - Give supplemental oxygen and monitor oxygen saturation
  - Give diphenhydramine 1 mg/kg intramuscularly
  - Give albuterol $\times$ 3 puffs
- Major:
  - Give epinephrine 0.01 mg/kg intramuscularly
  - Give diphenhydramine 1 mg/kg intramuscularly
  - Give dexamethasone 0.5 mg/kg intramuscularly
  - Administer CPR and call 911

Disposition:

- Minor allergic reactions may be treated with diphenhydramine and albuterol and resolve on their own. The patient should be referred for medical follow up.
- Major allergic reactions are life threatening; administer CPR if required, and call 911 for assistance and transport.

Approved by:_____ Date:_____

Uterine Hemorrhage Causing Hypotension

Description: Blood pressure is more than 20% below baseline. Hypotension can be associated with acute blood loss, prolonged fasting and dehydration, or allergic reactions to medications or systemic injection of local anesthetics. If hypotension is the result of uterine bleeding, immediate action must be taken.

Signs and Symptoms:

- Dizziness, light-headed feeling
- Nausea, vomiting
- Fever, dry mouth
- Excessive vaginal bleeding
- Rapid heart beat

Treatment:

- Place patient in supine position and elevate legs
- Give fluids as tolerated
- Start intravenous line and administer normal saline
- Identify site and attempt to stop source

Disposition:

- If the patient can slowly sit then stand without dizziness and bleeding has stopped, she may be discharged and given follow-up instructions and appointment.
- Evaluate the cervix and vagina to assess for laceration or etiology of vaginal bleeding. If bleeding is uterine in nature and is excessive, immediately transfer to the hospital for further treatment and evaluation must ensue.
- Administer CPR and call 911 if the patient has continued bleeding, loss of consciousness, or convulsions associated with low blood pressure.

Approved by:_____ Date:_____

Respiratory Arrest Caused by Laryngospasm

Description: Laryngospasm is a protective reflex preventing foreign material such as water, saliva, or foreign bodies from entering the lower airway. In patients who are awake, laryngospasm is usually brief followed by vigorous coughing. In sedated patients, laryngospasm can be more prolonged with less coughing.

Signs and Symptoms:

- Increased respiratory effort with difficulty in exchanging air
- Noisy respiration (crowing)
- Respiratory retractions: paradoxical inward movement of the chest with aspiratory effort

Treatment:
- Stop the procedure
- Place head down and turn to side
- Use fingers to clear airway of solid material and suction for liquid material
- Administer positive pressure oxygen by bag and mask
- Optimize the airway with head extension and jaw thrust
  —The pain produced by this maneuver will frequently break the laryngospasm
- If air exchange is not improving, call 911 for assistance

Disposition:

- Temporary oxygen desaturation during laryngospasm is common. The majority of patients will recover without problems. Oxygen saturation should return to pretreatment levels within 10 minutes.
- Persistent oxygen desaturation (less than 90% for over 10 minutes) may indicate aspiration of foreign material or, rarely, negative pressure pulmonary edema. Referral for immediate medical attention is indicated.
- Administer CPR and call 911 if laryngospasm is complicated by seizures or bradycardia (heart rate less than 60 in a child or less than 30 in an adult).

Approved by:_____ Date:_____

Excessive Sedation (Hypoventilation)

Description: Shallow, slow breathing results in inadequate removal of carbon dioxide (CO_2) from the lungs. This is usually caused by sedatives, which depress respiratory effort or can cause partial airway obstruction.

Signs and Symptoms:

- Early symptom is the sedated patient is unresponsive to deep painful stimulation
- Mild accumulation of CO_2 will stimulate respiration back toward normal levels and is usually asymptomatic
- Severe accumulation of CO_2 will result in oxygen desaturation and depression of respiratory effort. It may be associated with labored breathing, sweating, or somnolence.

Treatment:

- Decrease level of sedation (stop sedatives)
- Optimize airway with head extension and jaw thrust
  —The painful stimulus will increase respiration
- Provide oxygen supplement with bag and mask if necessary
- Monitor oxygen saturation
- Give reversal agents naxolone 0.4 mg (for narcotics) or flumazenil 0.2 mg (for midazolam or diazepam)

Disposition:

- Most cases of hypoventilation will resolve without problems if the airway is maintained.
- Administer CPR and call 911 if hypoventilation leads to loss of consciousness or apnea (no respiratory effort).

Approved by:_____ Date:_____

APPENDIX G-2

The Universal Patient Compact

Principles for Partnership

As your healthcare partner we pledge to:

- Include you as a member of the team
- Treat you with respect, honesty and compassion
- Always tell you the truth
- Include your family or advocate when you would like us to
- Hold ourselves to the highest quality and safety standards
- Be responsive and timely with our care and information to you
- Help you to set goals for your healthcare and treatment plans
- Listen to you and answer your questions
- Provide information to you in a way you can understand
- Respect your right to your own medical information
- Respect your privacy and the privacy of your medical information
- Communicate openly about benefits and risks associated with any treatments
- Provide you with information to help you make informed decisions about your care and treatment options
- Work with you, and other partners who treat you, in the coordination of your care

As a patient I pledge to:

- Be a responsible and active member of my healthcare team
- Treat you with respect, honesty and consideration
- Always tell you the truth
- Respect the commitment you have made to healthcare and healing
- Give you the information that you need to treat me
- Learn all that I can about my condition
- Participate in decisions about my care
- Understand my care plan to the best of my ability
- Tell you what medications I am taking
- Ask questions when I do not understand and until I do understand
- Communicate any problems I have with the plan for my care
- Tell you if something about my health changes
- Tell you if I have trouble reading
- Let you know if I have family, friends or an advocate to help me with my healthcare

---

© 2008 National Patient Safety Foundation. Used by permission.

APPENDIX G-3

Anesthesia

Anesthesia Contract Risks and Benefits

A significant element of office-based surgery is anesthesia. As described in the section on anesthesia, the level of anesthesia should be dictated by the type of procedure performed and the comfort of the patient. There is a wide range of options for anesthesia that may vary by patient, procedure, or both. There are many ways to deal with the complexity inherent in office-based surgery anesthesia, and all of them with the primary focus on patient preference, comfort, and safety. Some practices have found it to be advantageous to make use of a contract anesthesiologist. Following is a summary of the benefits and risks of this option.

Benefits

An advantage to having an anesthesia contract is that an anesthesiologist is able to devote full attention to the patient and the patient's anesthetic needs, while the surgeon is able to focus on the procedure.

An anesthesiologist has the ability to provide multiple levels of anesthesia during one procedure and for one patient if required. This allows for the variations in levels of sedation that may be required by different patients despite the procedure remaining unchanged. It would increase the percentage of patients who would be appropriate for office-based surgery. A contract with an anesthesiologist could include the anesthesiologist's responsibility for the individual patient, monitoring equipment (minimizing start-up and maintenance costs in the practice), medications, and requirement that staff remain up to date with mock drills. This is a model used in other specialties for office-based procedures and may be utilized based on an individual office and community needs and availability.

Risks

The guidelines for the performance of office-based surgery outlined in this document for the administration of moderate sedation anesthesia are adequate to ensure patient safety. The use of an anesthesiologist to administer that standard is not required. Retaining a contract anesthesiologist may have a financial impact on the cost of the office procedure. The availability and need for this relationship will vary based on individual needs, state rules and regulations, and health care provider preference. A contract relationship with an anesthesiologist is not available in every community. There are some health care providers who are able to provide a procedure and uphold excellence in patient safety standards while providing adequate anesthesia in a safe and patient-centered way.

(continued)

Continuum of Depth of Sedation
Definition of General Anesthesia and Levels of Sedation/Analgesia*

(Approved by ASA House of Delegates on October 13, 1999, and amended on October 27, 2004)

	Minimal Sedation (Anxiolysis)	Moderate Sedation/ Analgesia ("Conscious Sedation")	Deep Sedation/ Analgesia	General Anesthesia
Responsiveness	Normal response to verbal stimulation	Purposeful** response to verbal or tactile stimulation	Purposeful** response following repeated or painful stimulation	Unarousable even with painful stimulus
Airway	Unaffected	No intervention required	Intervention may be required	Intervention often required
Spontaneous Ventilation	Unaffected	Adequate	May be inadequate	Frequently inadequate
Cardiovascular Function	Unaffected	Usually maintained	Usually maintained	May be impaired

Minimal Sedation (Anxiolysis) is a drug-induced state during which patients respond normally to verbal commands. Although cognitive function and coordination may be impaired, ventilatory and cardiovascular functions are unaffected.

Moderate Sedation/Analgesia ("Conscious Sedation") is a drug-induced depression of consciousness during which patients respond purposefully** to verbal commands, either alone or accompanied by light tactile stimulation. No interventions are required to maintain a patent airway, and spontaneous ventilation is adequate. Cardiovascular function is usually maintained.

Deep Sedation/Analgesia is a drug-induced depression of consciousness during which patients cannot be easily aroused but respond purposefully** following repeated or painful stimulation. The ability to independently maintain ventilatory function may be impaired. Patients may require assistance in maintaining a patent airway, and spontaneous ventilation may be inadequate. Cardiovascular function is usually maintained.

General Anesthesia is a drug-induced loss of consciousness during which patients are not arousable, even by painful stimulation. The ability to independently maintain ventilatory function is often impaired. Patients often require assistance in maintaining a patent airway, and positive pressure ventilation may be required because of depressed spontaneous ventilation or drug-induced depression of neuromuscular function. Cardiovascular function may be impaired.

Because sedation is a continuum, it is not always possible to predict how an individual patient will respond. Hence, practitioners intending to produce a given level of sedation should be able to rescue*** patients whose level of sedation becomes deeper than initially intended. Individuals administering moderate sedation/analgesia ("conscious sedation") should be able to rescue*** patients who enter a state of deep sedation/analgesia, while those administering deep sedation/analgesia should be able to rescue*** patients who enter a state of general anesthesia.

*Monitored Anesthesia Care does not describe the continuum of depth of sedation, rather it describes "a specific anesthesia service in which an anesthesiologist has been requested to participate in the care of a patient undergoing a diagnostic or therapeutic procedure."

**Reflex withdrawal from a painful stimulus is NOT considered a purposeful response.

***Rescue of a patient from a deeper level of sedation than intended is an intervention by a practitioner proficient in airway management and advanced life support. The qualified practitioner corrects adverse physiologic consequences of the deeper-than-intended level of sedation (such as hypoventilation, hypoxia, and hypotension) and returns the patient to the originally intended level of sedation.

ASA Levels of Sedation, 2004, is reprinted with permission of the American Society of Anesthesiologists, 520 N. Northwest Highway, Park Ridge, Illinois, 600668-2573.

APPENDIX G-4

Sample Privileging Form

(sheet 1)

This sample application for privileges is provided for educational purposes only.
It may require modification for use in a particular facility.

Outpatient Privileging

Delineation for Privileges for:_____   Credentialing Period:_____

Practice Name:_____   Department:_____ Specialty:_____

Clinical Category	Procedure Description	Approximate Volume in Prior Year	Amount Required	Requested	Inpatient Privileges Y N N/A	Medical Director Approval Y N N/A
Cervix						
	LEEP	_____	_____	☐		
	Colposcopy cervix	_____	_____	☐		
	Laser therapy*	_____	_____	☐		
	Other:	_____	_____	☐		
Contraception						
	IUD insertion	_____	_____	☐		
	IUD removal	_____	_____	☐		
	Tubal ligation*	_____	_____	☐		
	Other:	_____	_____	☐		
Diagnostic Gyn ultrasound						
	Gyn U/S	_____	_____	☐		
	Sonohysteroscopy	_____	_____	☐		
	Other:	_____	_____	☐		
Diagnostic Ob ultrasound						
	3rd trimester OB U/S	_____	_____	☐		
	1st trimester OB U/S	_____	_____	☐		
	Other:	_____	_____	☐		
Excision of lesion						
	Excision of lesion trunk or exrm	_____	_____	☐		
	Excision of lesion genitalia	_____	_____	☐		
	Other:	_____	_____	☐		

Abbreviations: LEEP, loop electrosurgical excision procedure; IUD, intrauterine device; U/S, ultrasound; exrm, extremity.

*Denotes that procedure requires documentation of performance competency in an inpatient surgical setting prior to performing in an outpatient office setting.

Sample Privileging Form

(sheet 2)

Outpatient Privileging

Delineation for Privileges for:_____   **Credentialing Period:**_____

Practice Name:_____   **Department:**_____   **Specialty:**_____

Clinical Category	Procedure Description	Approximate Volume in Prior Year	Amount Required	Requested	Inpatient Privileges Y N N/A	Medical Director Approval Y N N/A
Needle aspiration						
	Needle aspiration of breast cyst	_____	_____	☐		
NST						
	Nonstress test	_____	_____	☐		
Pessary						
	Pessary fitting	_____	_____	☐		
Uterus						
	Endometrial biopsy	_____	_____	☐		
	D&C*	_____	_____	☐		
	Hysterosalpingogram	_____	_____	☐		
	Hysteroscopy*	_____	_____	☐		
	Ablation*	_____	_____	☐		
	Other:	_____	_____	☐		
Vagina						
	Destruction of vaginal lesion	_____	_____	☐		
	Vaginal biopsy	_____	_____	☐		
	Laser therapy*	_____	_____	☐		
	Colposcopy vagina*	_____	_____	☐		
	Other:	_____	_____	☐		
Vulvar						
	Destruction of vulva lesion	_____	_____	☐		
	Vulvar biopsy	_____	_____	☐		
	Laser therapy*	_____	_____	☐		
	Hymenotomy	_____	_____	☐		
	Perineoplasty	_____	_____	☐		
	I&D of vulva or perineal abscess	_____	_____	☐		
	Other:	_____	_____	☐		

Abbreviations: NST, nonstress test; D&C, dilation and curettage; I&D, incision and drainage.

*Denotes that procedure requires documentation of performance competency in an inpatient surgical setting prior to performing in an outpatient office setting.

APPENDIX G-5

Office Surgical Safety Checklist

How to Use the Office Surgical Safety Checklist

- Review the checklist with your entire office surgical team. Assign each task to the appropriate staff member (eg, patient's escort driver is confirmed by the front desk staff or the preoperative time-out is performed by the physician). This may vary from office to office.

- Assign one person (ie, physician or nurse) as checklist coordinator to be responsible for confirming the tasks on the list with the assigned individuals.

- The checklist coordinator should confirm each task verbally with the appropriate office team member to ensure the appropriate procedures have been implemented and documented. If necessary, the checklist coordinator also can obtain initials from each of the assigned individuals to confirm completion of their respective tasks.

- If the task does not apply to the patient, the checklist coordinator should confirm this with the physician (eg, the use of imaging may not apply to all patients).

- The checklist coordinator should stop the office surgery team from progressing to the next phase of the operation until all tasks have been appropriately addressed. Ideally, any team member should feel comfortable to stop the procedure if they have safety concerns.

- The office surgery team should debrief to discuss modifications for future uses of the checklist. Removing tasks is not recommended.

Office Surgical Safety Checklist

Patient Name: _____   Primary Diagnosis: _____   Date:_____

Date of Birth: _____   Procedure: _____

Preoperative (Before Anesthesia/Analgesia)

_____ ☐ Patient identity, site (marked), procedure, and consent confirmed

_____ ☐ Current history and physical on chart

_____ ☐ All medications taken previously that day reviewed and recorded

_____ ☐ Patient's escort driver confirmed

_____ ☐ No change in medical condition since last office visit, if changed, indicate here: _____

_____ ☐ *Nil per os* (nothing by mouth—NPO) status confirmed

_____ ☐ Preoperative instructions followed confirmed by patient

_____ ☐ Known allergies reviewed

_____ ☐ Any indicated lab work confirmed (eg, glucose level assessment in a diabetic patient or pregnancy test)

_____ ☐ Preoperative vital signs documented

_____ ☐ Pulse oximeter on the patient and functioning

_____ ☐ Airway or aspiration risk assessed

_____ ☐ Anesthesia and medication check is complete

_____ ☐ Essential imaging is displayed

Preoperative (Before Incision)

_____ ☐ Time-out (provider/patient/site/procedure)

_____ ☐ Antibiotic prophylaxis given within 60 minutes of incision

_____ ☐ Critical events anticipated:

_____ ☐ Critical or nonroutine steps   _____ ☐ How long case will take

_____ ☐ Anticipated blood loss   _____ ☐ Patient specific concerns

_____ ☐ Sterility   _____ ☐ Equipment issues

Intraoperative

_____ ☐ Intraoperative medications recorded

_____ ☐ If sedation implemented, oxygen saturation, blood pressure, pulse, and level of alertness monitored and documented every 5 minutes

_____ ☐ For hysteroscopic procedures:

_____ ☐ Cavity assessment recorded per manufacturer's guidelines

_____ ☐ Fluid balance documented

Postoperative

_____ ☐ Instrument, sponge, and needle counts completed

_____ ☐ Specimen labeling confirmed

_____ ☐ Equipment problems documented

_____ ☐ Key concerns for recovery and management of patient documented

Discharge

_____ ☐ Vital signs recorded and returned to within 20% of baseline

_____ ☐ Adequate level of consciousness, pain control, ability to tolerate liquids by mouth, and ability to void (if appropriate for the procedure) documented

_____ ☐ Discharge instruction sheet that includes how to recognize a postoperative emergency and steps to follow should one occur after discharge (eg, hemorrhage) discussed and given to patient

_____ ☐ Appropriate postoperative follow-up appointment scheduled

_____ ☐ Complications recorded

_____ ☐ Follow-up call 24–48 hours after procedure assigned

INDEX

Note: Page numbers followed by italicized letters *b*, *f*, or *t* indicate boxes, figures, and tables, respectively.

A

AAAHC. *See* Accreditation Association for Ambulatory Health Care
Abbreviations, Joint Commission "Do Not Use" list, 36–37, 36*t*
ABMS. *See* American Board of Medical Specialties
ABOG. *See* American Board of Obstetrics and Gynecology
Accreditation
  interrelationship with credentialing and privileging, 97
  and office-based practice, presidential task force findings on, 96–97
Accreditation Association for Ambulatory Health Care (AAAHC)
  contact information for, 79
  on peer review in ambulatory care settings, 52–53
Accreditation Council for Graduate Medical Education (ACGME)
  competencies, 10–11
  program requirements for surgical training, 33
ACGME. *See* Accreditation Council on Graduate Medical Education
Action plan, 71
ADE. *See* Adverse drug event
Adverse drug event (ADE). *See also* Medication error
  causes of, 56
  definition of, 71
  Prevention Study, 33
  rate of, 33, 56
Adverse events
  definition of, 37
  disclosure of, 37–39
    and apology, 37–38
    definition of, 37
    legal requirement for, 37
    and lowered litigation costs, 37–38
    and the second victim, 38–39
  postevent evaluation for, 10
  processing, institutional support in, 38–39
  professionals' response to, in residency education, 11
  root cause analysis, 67–70
  3Rs program for, 38
  trends in, analysis, 12
Adverse outcome index, 17, 18*t*
Agency for Healthcare Research and Quality (AHRQ)
  criteria for quality indicators, 16
  hospital safety survey tool, 28
  national organizations involved in performance measures, 80–81
  patient safety culture survey, 32
  survey on readiness for TeamSTEPPS, 32
AHRQ. *See* Agency for Healthcare Research and Quality
Allergic reactions, mock drill for, 100

AMA. *See* American Medical Association
Ambulatory Care Quality Alliance (AQA)
  contact information for, 79
  effort toward quality improvement, 51
  national organizations involved in performance measures, 82–83
American Board of Medical Specialties (ABMS), Maintenance of Certification program, 53
American Board of Obstetrics and Gynecology (ABOG), Maintenance of Certification program, 53–54
American College of Obstetricians and Gynecologists
  Committee on Patient Safety and Quality Improvement, 2
  opinion on abbreviation use, 37
  opinion on disclosure of adverse events, 37
  opinion on patient safety in surgical environment, 32
  policy on disclosure of adverse events, 37
  practice guidelines, 14
American Medical Association (AMA)
  national organizations involved in performance measures, 86–87
  Physician Consortium for Performance Improvement, 91
Analgesia, levels of, 104
Anesthesia, in office-based surgery, 94, 103–104
AQA. *See* Ambulatory Care Quality Alliance

B

Barcode, 34
Bell-shaped curve, 59, 60*f*
Benchmark, 16
  definition of, 71
  resources for, 79
Briefing
  definition of, 71
  meetings for, 26
  safety, 23–24
Brown bag prescription bottle checks, 56

C

CAHPS. *See* Hospital Consumer Assessment of Healthcare Providers and Systems Hospital Survey
Call out, 31
Cause and effect diagram, 62, 62*f*
Centers for Medicare and Medicaid Services (CMS), 2, 82–83
Certificate renewal, 53
Certification
  board, of credentialing and privileging, 44
  maintenance of, 53
Change initiatives, steps in, 25
Chart review, 19, 20–21, 22*f*
Check-back, 31
Checklists
  for data collection and measurement, 14*b*
  high reliability organizations and, 5
  hospital surgical safety, 88
  for office-based practice, 92–93, 107–108

Clinical pathways
  definition of, 71
  development of, 13–14
Clinical protocols, 25
CMS. *See* Centers for Medicare and Medicaid Services
Committee on Patient Safety and Quality Improvement, 2
Communication
  and changing physician behavior, 24–25
  closed loop, 31
  electronic, 27
  failures, and sentinel events, 31
  and improved patient safety, 29–30
  in outpatient settings, 54–55, 57
  and patient safety, 56, 57
  strategies for, 31–32
  in surgical environment, 33
Communication skills, in residency training, 10, 11
Competencies, Accreditation Council for Graduate Medical Education, 10–11
Computerized Physician Order Entry (CPOE), 34, 71–72
Construct validity, 72
Continuous quality improvement, 12–13, 72
Control chart, 61, 61*f*
CPOE. *See* Computerized Physician Order Entry
Credentialing
  definition of, 43, 72
  department chair's role in, 11
  for family physicians, 47–48
  interrelationship with privileging and accreditation, 97
  and office-based practice, presidential task force findings on, 95–96
  process of, 43
  reappraisal, prerequisites for, 44

D

Data analysis
  clinical example, 63
  tools for, 59–63
Data collection and measurement, 18
  checklist for, 14*b*
  planning for, 14*b*
Debriefings, 10, 71
Department of obstetrics and gynecology
  in academic setting, chair, leadership responsibilities of, 10–11
  chair, roles and responsibilities of, 8–9
  information sharing in, 27
  leadership, and quality improvement, 7–11
  meetings
    agenda for, 26
    chairing, 26
    effective, strategies for, 26–27
    facilitating, 26
    management of, 26
    and system improvement, 25–26
  in nonacademic setting, chair, leadership responsibilities of, 8–9
  quality improvement committee, 8

Discharge summary, importance of, 57
Disruptive behavior
    definition of, 72
    by physician, 22–23
Due process
    definition of, 72
    during stages of corrective actions, 22

E
Electronic administration technology
        (eMAR), 34
Electronic health record, 34
Electronic prescribing, 34
eMAR. *See* Electronic administration
        technology
Errors. *See also* Adverse events; Medication
        errors
    definition of, 72
    human, systems approaches to, 3–4
    medical
        Institute of Medicine report on, 2–3
        reduction, strategies for, 5
        risk factors for, 4
Evidence-based clinical indicators, 16
Evidence-based guidelines, 2, 2f

F
Face validity
    definition of, 72
    for quality indicators, 16
Facilitator, 26, 67–68, 72
Failure, preoccupation with, 4, 7
Failure Mode and Effects Analysis (FMEA),
        65–67, 66f
Family-centered care, 55–56
Family physicians
    credentialing for, 47–48
    gynecologic privileges for, 48
    obstetric privileges for, 47–48
Ferrari race team, teamwork skills of, 30
Fishbone diagram, 62, 62f, 68, 68f
Five Rights of Medication Use, 34, 72
FMEA. *See* Failure Mode and Effects
        Analysis
Focused professional practice evaluation, 19
Forcing functions, 5, 72

G
General anesthesia, 104
Gloves, in inpatient setting, 35–36
Guidelines, and quality of care, 14–15

H
Hand hygiene, in inpatient setting, 35–36
Handoffs, execution of, in residency
        education, 11
HCAHPS. *See* Hospital Consumer
        Assessment of Healthcare Providers
        and Systems
Healthcare Effectiveness Data and
        Information Set (HEDIS), 51, 79
Health Care Quality Improvement Act, 18–19
Health care, Institute of Medicine
        recommendations for advances in
        U.S., 2–3
Health literacy, 54–55, 72
HEDIS. *See* Healthcare Effectiveness Data
        and Information Set
High reliability organizations (HROs)
    characteristics, 4–5, 7, 9
    definition of, 73

Histogram, 61–62, 61f
Hospital Consumer Assessment of
        Healthcare Providers and Systems
        (HCAHPS), 28–29
Hospital Quality Alliance (HQA), 84–85
Hospital surgical safety checklist, 88
HQA. *See* Hospital Quality Alliance
HROs. *See* High reliability organizations

I
Idealized Design of Perinatal Care, 25
Indicator. *See also* Quality indicators, 73
Infections, nosocomial, mortality rate for, 35
Infection control, 35–36
Information technology systems
    and medication safety, 34
    in outpatient settings, 57
Informed consent, 33, 73, 93–94
Informed decision making, 73
Innovation, clinical, 2, 2f
Inpatient setting
    institutional models, 7
    quality improvement and patient safety
        in, 7–42
Institute of Medicine (IOM)
    aims for quality improvement, 16
    *Crossing the Quality Chasm: A New
        Health System for the 21st Century*,
        2–3, 16
    *To Err is Human: Building a Safer Health
        System*, 2–3
    *Medicare: A Strategy for Quality
        Assurance*, 2, 17–18
Intravenous (IV) medication administration,
        smart technology and, 34
IOM. *See* Institute of Medicine
Ishikawa diagram, 62, 62f
IV medication administration. *See*
        Intravenous medication
        administration

J
JCAHO. *See* Joint Commission on
        Accreditation of Healthcare
        Organizations
Job satisfaction, improved, teams and, 32
Joint Commission, 1, 79
    on adverse events, 29–30
    on causes of sentinel events, 31
    contact information for, 72
    "Do Not Use" list of abbreviations,
        36–37, 36t
    hand hygiene requirements, 35
    medication reconciliation requirement, 35
    national organizations involved in
        performance measures, 84–85
    on peer review in ambulatory care
        settings, 52
    position paper on wrong site surgery, 32
    requirement for disclosure of adverse
        events, 37, 38
    requirement for root cause analysis, 69–70
    Sentinel Event Alert, 29–30
    sentinel event policy, 69–70
    Universal Protocol for Preventing Wrong
        Site, Wrong Procedure, and Wrong
        Person Surgery, 32–33
Joint Commission on Accreditation of
        Healthcare Organizations (JCAHO).
        See Joint Commission
Just culture, 73

L
Larygnospam, respiratory arrest caused by,
        mock drill for, 101
Leadership
    definition of, 7
    departmental, 7–8
    effective, characteristics needed for, 9
    in quality improvement, 7–11
    roles and responsibilities for, 8
    styles, 8
Lean, 64–65
Leapfrog Group, 84–85
Local anesthetic toxicity, mock drill for,
        99–100

M
Maintenance of Certification (MOC), 53–54
Managing Obstetrical Risk Efficiently
        (MORE^OB) program, 25
Mean, 59
Measures. *See* Quality indicators
Median, 59
Medical errors. *See* Adverse events; Errors,
        medical
Medical records. *See also* Electronic health
        record
    review, 20–21, 22f
    screening, 19–20
Medication errors
    in inpatient setting
        costs of, 33–34
        prevention of, 34–35
        rate of, 33
        ordering and, 34–35
    in outpatient settings
        prevention of, 56
        sources of, 56
Medication reconciliation, 35
Medication safety
    Five Rights of Medication Use and, 34, 72
    information technology and, 34
    in inpatient setting, 33–35
    in outpatient settings, 56
    patient education and, 35
    in surgical environment, 33
Meetings. *See also* Department of obstetrics
        and gynecology, meetings
    for briefing, 26
    management of, 26
    for negotiation, 26
    parliamentary, 26
    for problem solving, 26
    types of, 26
Methicillin-resistant *Staphylococcus aureus*
        (MRSA) infection, prevention, 35–36
MOC. *See* Maintenance of Certification
Mock drills, 93, 99–101
Mode, 59
Morbidity and mortality conferences, 10
MORE^OB program. *See* Managing Obstetrical
        Risk Efficiently program
MRSA. *See* Methicillin-resistant
        Staphylococcus aureus infection
Myocardial infarction, mock drill for, 100

N
National Committee for Quality Assurance
        (NCQA)
    contact information for, 79
    development of HEDIS by, 51
    national organizations involved in
        performance measures, 84–85

National Perinatal Information Center/ Quality Analytics Service, 79
National Quality Forum (NQF)
    contact information for, 79
    national organizations involved in performance measures, 86–87
National Practitioner Data Bank, 19, 22, 43
National Quality Measures Clearinghouse (NQMC), 79
NCQA. *See* National Committee for Quality Assurance
Near misses
    definition of, 37, 73
    postevent evaluation for, 10
    root cause analysis, 67–70

O

Office-based practice. *See also* Outpatient setting
    and accreditation, presidential task force findings on, 96–97
    and anesthesia, 94, 103–104
    checklists for, 92–93, 107–108
    and credentialing, presidential task force findings on, 95–96
    emergency medication in, 95
    excessive sedation in, patient rescue from, 95
    informed consent process for, 93–94
    medical director of, 91–92
    mock drills in, 93, 99–101
    patient information in, 95
    and patient rights and responsibilities, 94
    patient safety in, report of presidential task force on, 91–98
    policy and procedure manual for, 93
    and privileging, presidential task force findings on, 96
    procedure outcome reporting system for, 94–95
    procedures and equipment used in, industry and, 97–98
    resuscitative policy in, 95
    time-outs in, 95
Office of Communications and Knowledge Transfer, 79
Office surgical safety checklist, 92–93, 107–108
Opportunity statements, 12
Outcomes
    definition of, 74
    follow-up and, 57
    improved, teams and, 32
    patient adherence to follow-up plans and, 57
    reporting system, for office-based practice, 94–95
    unanticipated, disclosure of, 37–38
Outliers
    definition of, 74
    identifying, 1, 20, 21
Outpatient setting
    coordination of care in, 57
    effectiveness-of-care measures for, 51
    follow-up care in, 57
    performance measurement system for, development of, 52
    quality improvement and patient safety in, 51–58
    transition from hospital to, 57

P

Pareto chart, 62–63, 63*f*
Patient-centered care, 11, 55–56
Patient education
    and medication safety, 35
    teach-back method, 55, 56
Patient health literacy. *See* Health literacy
Patient rights and responsibilities, 94
Patients, partnering with, 55–56, 102
Patient safety. *See also* Safety culture
    culture of, 24
    definition of, 74
    in inpatient settings, 7–42
    Institute of Medicine recommendations on, 2–3
    in office setting, report of presidential task force on, 91–98
    in outpatient settings, 51–58, 91–98
    and procedures and equipment used in office-based setting, 97–98
    report of presidential task force on, 91–98
    program, in inpatient setting, elements of, 27–29
    in surgical environment, 32–33
    systems approaches to, 3–4
Patient safety leader, 24
Patient safety leadership WalkRounds, 23
Patient satisfaction, assessment of, 28–29
PDSA cycle. *See* Plan–Do–Study–Act cycle
Peer review, 18–19, 26
    and acceptable variations, 21
    and deficiencies in care, 21
    definition of, 52
    instruments for, 19
    in outpatient and office settings, 52–53
    process for, 19
Performance
    knowledge-based, 4
    rule-based, 4
    skill-based, 4
Performance measurement
    continuous monitoring and, 19
    data for, 18
    national organizations involved in performance measures, 80–87
    for outpatient, ambulatory, and small practice settings, 52, 52*b*
    in small facilities, 19*b*
Performance measures, 17–18
    advantages of, 18
    definition of, 74
    outcomes-based, 18
    for outpatient, ambulatory, and small practice settings, 52, 52*b*
    process-based, 18
    types of, 18–19
Perinatal safety programs, 25, 29–30
Physician. *See also* Family physicians
    delivering deficient care, and corrective actions by department, 21–22
    disruptive behavior by, 22–23, 72
    effect of medical errors on, 38–39
    impairment, 22–23, 74
    involvement in quality improvement and patient safety, 23
    in office-based practice
        performance measures and reporting requirements for, 51
        and quality improvement, 51

Physician (*continued*)
    reentry
        definition of, 48
        and recredentialing and reprivileging, 11, 48–49
        responsibility for quality improvement, 51
Physician behavior, changing, 24–25
Physician champions, 24
Physician Consortium for Performance Improvement, 79, 86–87
Physician Quality Reporting Initiative, 79
Physician Reentry Program (PREP), 49
Plan–Do–Study–Act (PDSA) cycle, 63–64, 64*f*, 74
Postevent evaluation, 10
Practice guidelines. *See* American College of Obstetricians and Gynecologists, practice guidelines
Preceptorship, 48, 74
PREP. *See* Physician Reentry Program
Presidential Task Force on Patient Safety in the Office Setting, report of, 91–98
Privileges and privileging
    after period of inactivity, 11, 48–49
    application for, sample form, 105–106
    criteria for, 43
    core, 43
    definition of, 74
    department chair's role in, 11
    granting, 43–44
    prerequisites for, 43–44
    gynecologic
        for family physicians, 48
        level I, 44–45
        level II, 45
        level III-A, basic endoscopic, 45
        level III-B, advanced endoscopic, 45–46
        level III-C, gynecologic oncology, 46
        level III-D, assisted reproductive technologies, 46
        level III-E, laser therapy, 46
        level III-F, endometrial ablation, 46–47
    interrelationship with credentialing and accreditation, 97
    levels of privileges for, 43
    new, requests for, 48–49
    for new equipment, 48
    for new technologies, 43, 48
    obstetric
        for family physicians, 47–48
        level I, 44
        level II, 44
        level III, 44
    and office-based practice, presidential task force findings on, 91–96
    procedures permitted under, 43
    process of, 43
    quality indicators and, 16
    reappraisal, prerequisites for, 44
Process, 74
Process improvement teams, 24
Proctoring, 44, 47, 48, 49, 74
Professionalism, in residency education, 11

Q

Quality assessment
    Donabedian model, 1
    measurement tools for, 63–70

Quality assessment (continued)
  outcomes in, 1
  process in, 1
  structure in, 1
Quality assurance, historical perspective
  on, 1
Quality improvement
  aims for, 2
  basic approach to, 13–15
  clinical innovation in, 2, 2f
  clinical strategies for, 1–2, 2f
  continuous, 1–2, 2f, 12–13, 72
  definition of, 74
  departmental program for, development
    of, 12–13
  educational approach for, 12, 13t
  graduate medical education on, 10
  historical perspective on, 1
  in inpatient settings, 7–42
  leadership in, 7–11
  in outpatient settings, 51–58
  projects, 12, 13t
  review process in, 8
Quality improvement committee
  decision on chart review, 20–21
  and deficiencies in care, 21
  departmental, 8
  and performance profiles, 21
  residents' participation on, 10
Quality indicators, 15–17
  criteria for, 16
  definition of, 15
  evidence-based, 16
  as monitors of sentinel events, 16
  nationally accepted or standardized, 17
  outcomes, 15, 17t, 18
  process, 15–16, 18
  rate-based, 16
  thresholds for, 16–17
  and trending, 16
  use of, pros and cons, 15b
Quality measurement, tools for, 63–70
QualityNet, 79
Quality of care
  concerns about, addressing, in inpatient
    setting, 21–23
  definition of, 2

R
RCA. See Root cause analysis
Read-backs, 35, 74
Recertification, voluntary, 53
Recredentialing, 11, 48–49, 74
Reentry
  definition of, 48
  recredentialing and reprivileging for, 11,
    48–49
  skills assessment for, 48–49
Reminder systems, in outpatient settings,
  56–57
Reprivileging, 11, 48–49
Residency training programs, and reentry,
  49
Residents
  competencies, 10–11
  didactic education of, safety and quality
    improvement incorporated into,
    10–11

Residents (continued)
  effect of medical errors on, 38–39
  experiential education of, safety and
    quality improvement incorporated
    into, 11
  safety principles and practices taught
    to, 10
Resources, for measure specifications,
  standards, or benchmarks, 79
Respiratory arrest, caused by laryngospasm,
  mock drill, 101
Root cause analysis (RCA), 67–70
  development of, template for, 68–69, 69f
  regulatory requirements for, 69–70
  team for, 67–68
3Rs program, for adverse events, 38
Run chart, 59–61, 60f

S
Safety. See also Medication safety; Patient
    safety
  graduate medical education on, 10
  targeted training in, 5
Safety attitudes questionnaire, 27–28
Safety briefings, 23–24
Safety culture
  creating, 9, 29, 29b
  definition of, 74–75
  elements of, 27
  and medication safety, 34
Safety survey
  examples, 28
  in inpatient setting, 27–28
SBAR. See Situation–Background–
    Assessment–Recovery
SD. See Standard deviation
Second Victim, 38–39
Sedation
  depth, 104
  excessive
    mock drill for, 101
    patient rescue from, in office-based
      practice, 95
Sentinel events
  causes of, 31
  definition of, 75
  Joint Commission policy on, 69–70
  quality indicators as monitors of, 16
  root cause analysis of, 67–70
Shared medical decision making, 33, 75
Sharp end, 3, 75
Simulation centers, and reentry, 49
Situation–Background–Assessment–
    Recovery (SBAR), 31–32
Six Sigma, 64–65
Standard deviation (SD), 59, 60f
Standardization, and care quality, 5
Standards
  and quality of care, 14
  resources for, 79
Statistical variation, 59
Structure–Process–Outcome triad, 75
Surgery, wrong site, 32–33
Surgical environment, patient safety in,
  32–33
Surveys
  of health care team, on safety, 27–28
  patient satisfaction, 28–29

Swiss cheese model of system accidents, 3,
  4f, 75

T
Teach-back, 55, 56
Teams. See also Teamwork
  medical
    benefits of, 32
    communication among, 31
    core, 30
    explicit, 30
    functions of, 30–32
    implementation of, 32
    implicit, 30
    leadership of, 31
    and multiteam environments, 30
    and mutual support, 31
    and situation monitoring, 31
    structure of, 30
  for quality improvement project,
    12–13
  root cause analysis, 67–68
TeamSTEPPS, 10–11, 32
Team training principles, in residency
  education, 10–11
Teamwork. See also Teams
  and error prevention, 29
  Ferrari race team's skills at, 30
  implementation, barriers to, 30
  medical
    implementation of, 32
    and improved patient safety, 29–30
  in residency education, 11
Threshold, 21, 75–76
Time-outs, 32
  definition of, 76
  in office-based surgery, 95
Tools
  for data analysis, 59–63
  for quality measurement, 63–70
Tracking systems, in outpatient settings,
  56–57
Trending, 16, 21
Two-challenge rule, 31

U
Unanticipated events, postevent evaluation
  for, 10
Universal Patient Compact, 102
Universal Protocol for Preventing Wrong
  Site, Wrong Procedure, and Wrong
  Person Surgery, 32–33
Uterine hemorrhage and hypotension, mock
  drill for, 100–101

V
Variation
  common cause, 59
  special cause, 59
Vasovagal episode, mock drill for, 99
Voluntary Review of Quality of Care
  (VRQC), 14, 25, 77
VRQC. See Voluntary Review of Quality of
  Care

W
WalkRounds, 23
Workaround, 76